Biomedical Materials for Multi-functional Applications

Series Editors

Arnab Chanda, Centre for Biomedical Engineering, Indian Institute of Technology Delhi, New Delhi, Germany

Sarabjeet Sidhu, Department of Mechanical Engineering, Sardar Beant Singh State University, Gurdaspur, UK

The series 'Biomedical Materials for Multi-functional Applications' is intended for the audience with an interest in biomaterials for various applications, including bio-implants, bio-instrumentation, biomechanics, and tissue engineering. The book titles under this series will bring different areas of biomedical engineering, bioengineering, materials science, mechanical engineering, and biosciences under one umbrella of biomedical materials. The books in this series will provide deep insights into the state-of-art of biomedical materials and deal with diverse and interdisciplinary aspects of biomaterials, ranging from basic science to host responses, as well as real-time applications. Some of the topics include but are not limited to: functional materials, smart materials, biomimetic materials, polymers, composites, ceramics, metals, alloys, and nanomaterials. This series will provide the most recent advances in biomedical materials, including design, synthesis, processing, and characterization. This series will accept both authored and edited volumes, including monographs, textbooks, reference works, and handbooks. This series aims to publish new advances in biomedical materials that have been made in the fabrication and development of biomaterials for different applications and the advancement of principles, theories, and designs. Each book title in the series will give a comprehensive overview of pioneering topics, and the readers will gain new knowledge and insights about the topic. As a collection, the series on 'Biomedical Materials for Multi-functional Applications' is anticipated to benefit a wide audience in academia, the research community, and industry.

Arnab Chanda · Gurpreet Singh

Diabetic Foot Ulcer

Characterization and Mitigation

Springer

Arnab Chanda
Centre for Biomedical Engineering
Indian Institute of Technology Delhi
New Delhi, Delhi, India

Gurpreet Singh
Centre for Biomedical Engineering
Indian Institute of Technology Delhi
New Delhi, Delhi, India

ISSN 2731-9695 ISSN 2731-9709 (electronic)
Biomedical Materials for Multi-functional Applications
ISBN 978-981-95-2483-9 ISBN 978-981-95-2484-6 (eBook)
https://doi.org/10.1007/978-981-95-2484-6

This Springer imprint is published by the registered company Springer Nature Singapore Pte Ltd.
The registered company address is: 152 Beach Road, #21-01/04 Gateway East, Singapore 189721, Singapore

Preface

Diabetic foot ulcers are one of the major complications of chronic diabetes mellitus, especially among the older population. Peripheral arterial disorder, peripheral neuropathy (loss of sensation), and irregular pressure loading of the plantar region cause foot ulcers. Foot ulcers not only hinder one's mobility but may also grow over time or cause additional ulcer formations in the absence of normal healing in diabetic patients and, in some severe cases, also lead to amputations. The diabetic ulcers have been studied widely in medical literature, but their accurate structural and mechanical impact when they appear on the foot has limited understanding. To date, there is no literature on the biomechanical modeling of a detailed diabetic foot to investigate diabetic ulceration with varying sizes, shapes, and depths. This monograph focuses on the characterization and mitigation of diabetic foot ulcers. India is one of the top healthcare providers in the world and has 101 million diabetic and 136 million prediabetic patients. Therefore, this work on the biomechanical modeling of diabetic ulcers will provide novel insights into diabetic foot ulceration, its progression, and management using plantar pressure offloading (insoles).

Chapter 1 of this book presents a detailed background of diabetes, diabetic foot, and ulceration development, emphasizing the pathophysiology and principles of management of the diabetic foot. This chapter discusses the motivation, significance, problem statement, and research gap in the biomechanical modeling and management of diabetic foot ulcers. Chapter 2 provides an overview of diabetic foot complications and ulceration. This chapter covers the biomechanics of foot structure, plantar pressure distribution, and a detailed review of the existing computational models for diabetic foot ulcers. Chapter 3 focuses on the biomechanical modeling of diabetic ulcers in different foot types. Computational models of both normal foot and flatfoot were developed and simulated with varying ulcer diameters and depths to quantify plantar stresses and assess ulcer risks across these foot types. Building on this work, Chap. 4 explores the biomechanical modeling of diabetic ulcers across all possible locations on the foot. The results were analyzed in terms of pressure distribution and ulcer risk at each location, with a discussion on the implications of ulcer location for clinical interventions. Chapter 5 presents a new finite element modeling method to analyze realistic wound shapes and the stresses involved during healing.

This research goes beyond standard wound types to examine diabetic, venous, pressure, and ulcer wounds while considering natural skin tension across healing phases. The findings offer important insights for pre-surgical planning and robotic-assisted wound closure, helping to prevent tissue overstrain and enhance healing outcomes.

Chapter 6 emphasizes the imperative need for ongoing technological advancements within the field with the overarching goal of improving patient outcomes and mitigating the complications associated with diabetic foot conditions. Also, various medical interventions and clinical practices used for the treatment of diabetic foot ulcers were discussed to find the research gaps and technological advancements needed in this area. Chapter 7 details the development of a smart pressure measurement insole designed to measure the plantar pressure values and a modular insole for plantar pressure offloading. It provides an in-depth discussion of the pressure measurement insole's design, sensor integration, functionality, and validation. Chapter 8 focuses on the design concept and rationale behind the development of the modular insole. Its effectiveness was validated through a comparative study involving two groups: 15 healthy participants and 15 diabetic participants. This study demonstrated the efficacy of the modular insole using experimental results. Finally, Chap. 9 summarizes the key findings of the work, highlighting their implications for diabetic foot management, clinical practice, patient care, and scientific research. Additionally, it outlines the limitations, potential directions for future investigations, and clinical applications. The findings of the work present important information on the foot condition post-ulceration and may help identify possibilities of further ulceration in the diabetic foot. In addition, the findings are anticipated to be indispensable for developing suitable interventions (e.g., custom orthotics) for diabetic foot ulcer management.

New Delhi, India
May 2025

Arnab Chanda
arnab.chanda@cbme.iitd.ac.in

Gurpreet Singh
gurpreet.singh@cbme.iitd.ac.in

Competing Interests The authors have no competing interests to declare that are relevant to the content of this manuscript.

Contents

About the Authors

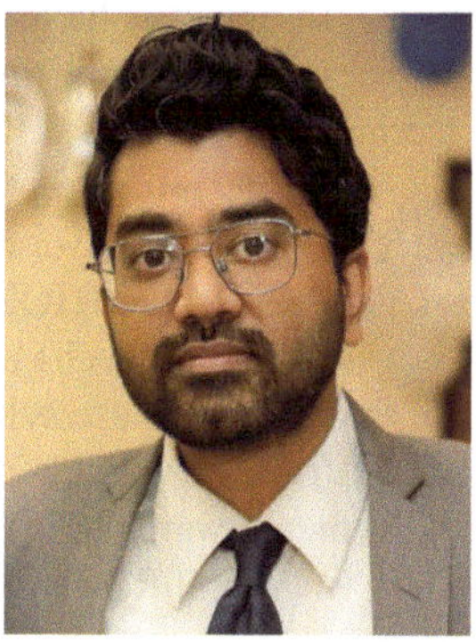

Arnab Chanda is an Associate Professor at the Centre for Biomedical Engineering, Indian Institute of Technology (IIT) Delhi, and a joint faculty at the Department of Biomedical Engineering, AIIMS, Delhi. He is also the founder of a start-up company, BIOFIT Technologies LLC, USA. He earned his Ph.D. from the University of Alabama, USA, and worked as a postdoctoral researcher at the University of Pittsburgh, USA. Dr. Chanda is an expert in the area of "Biomechanics", especially in tissue mimicking (artificial tissues) and characterization, finite element modeling (FEM), robotics and wearable device development, and entrepreneurship. He has been the recipient of various awards, including the Young Researcher Award and Early Career Award from ASME, MHRD, and AO Spine International-Singapore, and Top-Cited Paper Awards from IOP Publishing and Wiley. He holds and has filed 10+ US and Indian Patents, authored multiple Books and 100+ articles in reputed international journals. He is also the Coordinator of two successful Executive Programs: "Executive Program in Healthcare Entrepreneurship and Management" and "Executive Program in Robotics", Online PG Diploma in Healthcare Product Development and Management, and multiple Swayam/NPTEL courses for engineers, doctors, and management professionals. Dr. Chanda currently serves as the Associate Editor for the Journal of Appl. Biomaterials and Func. Materials, Book Series Editor for "Biomedical Materials for Multi-functional Applications", published by Springer Nature, Editorial Board Member for Nature Scientific Reports, and guest editor for several journals.

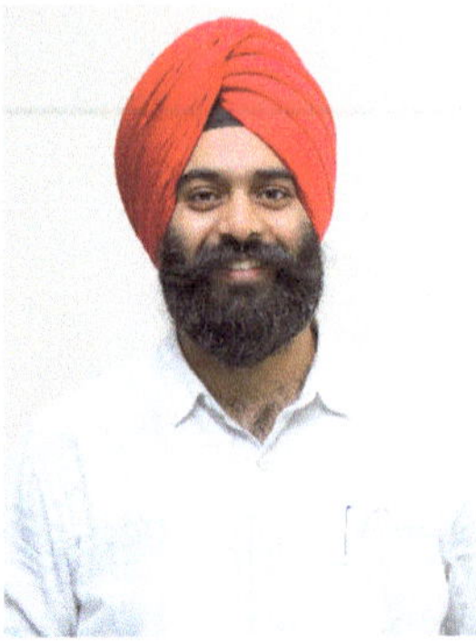

Gurpreet Singh is currently an Early-Doc Fellow at the Indian Institute of Technology (IIT) Delhi, where he completed his Ph.D. in Biomedical Engineering as a Prime Minister's Research Fellow (PMRF). His interdisciplinary research spans biomimetics, soft tissue mechanics, artificial tissue development, computational biomechanics, and medical intervention design. During his Ph.D., he developed biomechanical models for diabetic foot ulcers and designed a modular insole for pressure offloading. He has also worked on developing artificial tissue surrogates and computational models of brain aneurysms, integrating experimental and simulation approaches. Previously, during his M.Tech., he worked on surface modification of metallic biomaterials using electro-discharge machining to enhance bioactivity. He has contributed to 50+ peer-reviewed publications and book chapters in international journals and conferences. He has also authored some monograph books and co-edited a volume. He has received several recognitions, including the Top Cited Paper Award (IOP Publishing 2023) for his review article on the mechanical properties of soft human tissues, the Research Excellence Travel Award (RETA) from IIT Delhi in 2024, the Dogra Educational Endowment Award (2025), and nomination for the Amit Garg Memorial Research Excellence Award. He is serving as a reviewer for leading international journals.

Nomenclature

3D	Three-dimensional
AZP	Average Zonal Pressure
CAD	Computer Aided Design
CAGR	Compound Annual Growth Rate
CMI	Custom-Made Insole
CT	Computed Tomography
DFUs	Diabetic Foot Ulcers
DM	Diabetes Mellitus
DP	Diabetic Participants
FE	Finite Element
FEA	Finite Element Analysis
FEM	Finite Element Modeling
FSR	Force-Sensitive Resistors
HP	Healthy Participants
IDE	Integrated Development Environment
IDF	International Diabetes Federation
kPa	Kilopascal
MPa	Megapascal
MRI	Magnetic Resonance Imaging
PCA	Principal Component Analysis
RCW	Removable Cast Walker
S.D.	Standard Deviation
TCC	Total Contact Cast
TPU	Thermoplastic Polyurethane

Chapter 1
Introduction

1.1 Background and Motivation for the Study

Diabetes mellitus (DM) is a chronic and noncommunicable disease that poses a significant public health challenge across the globe. According to the International Diabetes Federation (IDF), approximately 536 million adults between the ages of 20 and 79 are currently living with diabetes in India. This figure is especially concerning, as projections indicate that the number of affected individuals could rise to 645 million by 2030 and may reach an alarming 784 million by 2045 if current trends persist [1]. The complications arising from diabetes are multifaceted and can severely diminish an individual's quality of life. Among the most common complications are diabetic ketoacidosis, a serious condition that can be life-threatening without prompt medical attention, and neuropathy, which involves nerve damage that can lead to a loss of sensation in the extremities [2, 3]. Other serious complications include hypoglycemia (dangerously low blood sugar levels), mastopathy (changes in breast tissue), and a variety of kidney-related diseases, alongside cardiovascular issues that significantly increase the risk of heart attacks and strokes. Additionally, diabetic retinopathy can severely impair vision and increase the risk of blindness, while hyperosmolar acidosis represents another critical condition that requires urgent care. Musculoskeletal disorders are also prevalent, further complicating the health landscape for individuals with diabetes. Among the various complications, diabetic foot ulcers (DFUs) are particularly concerning due to their increasing incidence and severity [4, 5]. This rise can be attributed not only to the growing number of diabetes cases but also to advancements in medical treatments that have extended the lives of individuals with diabetes, increasing the likelihood of complications. DFUs are especially troubling because they can lead to serious infections, limb amputations, and, in severe cases, death if not managed appropriately and swiftly. Timely intervention and proactive care are essential in addressing DFUs to prevent these dire outcomes and improve the overall health and well-being of individuals living with diabetes [6, 7].

A. Chanda and G. Singh, *Diabetic Foot Ulcer*, Biomedical Materials for Multi-functional Applications, https://doi.org/10.1007/978-981-95-2484-6_1

In low- and middle-income countries, several critical factors amplify the burden of foot diseases among patients with diabetes. One significant concern is the prevalent practice of walking barefoot, which increases the risk of traumatic injuries, infections, and foot ulcers. Many individuals lack awareness about proper foot care practices, including daily inspection, cleansing, and the use of suitable footwear, which are essential for preventing complications. Additionally, there's often a cultural stigma surrounding foot problems that discourages timely consultations with healthcare professionals, leading to delays in seeking necessary medical attention for foot issues. Further complicating the situation is the shortage of trained healthcare providers and specialized foot care services, which are crucial in appropriately managing diabetic foot conditions [8]. Research indicates that the global prevalence of foot ulceration among diabetics ranges from 1.7% to 6.3%, with a staggering 25% of individuals diagnosed with diabetes likely to experience foot ulceration during their lifetime. This data highlights the urgent need for a multifaceted approach that includes increased awareness, comprehensive education, and resource allocation focused on prevention and management strategies. To effectively combat DFUs, targeted interventions should be implemented, particularly in vulnerable populations where the risks are highest [9, 10]. Enhanced community health education initiatives could inform patients about the importance of foot hygiene and routine check-ups. Moreover, integrating training programs for healthcare providers would ensure that they possess the skills necessary to deliver proper foot care and promptly address complications. By employing these strategies, we could significantly reduce the incidence of DFUs and improve overall health outcomes for individuals living with diabetes, ultimately alleviating the substantial burden that foot diseases impose on both patients and healthcare systems [11–13].

The initial injury that leads to DFUs can arise from several sources, including acute mechanical trauma, thermal injuries, or cumulative repetitive stress placed on the feet over time. Individuals with diabetes, especially those experiencing peripheral neuropathy, often have a diminished ability to perceive pain, heat, or pressure in their extremities. This condition significantly increases the risk of unnoticed injuries, as minor traumas, such as friction from ill-fitting shoes, small cuts, or abrasions, are frequently overlooked [14–17]. The loss of protective sensation due to neuropathy can cause even trivial injuries to escalate unchecked, leading to more severe complications. Such injuries can result in the breakdown of the soft skin on the plantar surface of the foot, leading to the development of painful and potentially serious ulcers [18–22]. DFUs cause significant biomechanical changes associated with diabetes, which can impair the body's natural healing processes. Many patients struggle to recognize the severity of minor wounds or cuts, often misattributing pain or discomfort to other factors, which can lead to a dangerous delay in seeking appropriate medical care. This delay can have dire consequences as diabetic wounds are typically slow to heal and can be challenging to manage effectively, ultimately increasing the risk of complications [18–20]. What starts as a minor deformity or skin irritation can swiftly progress into a serious ulceration, which usually has a low probability of healing without timely and appropriate intervention. The financial burden of treating DFUs is considerable; these ulcers account for as much as 33% of all healthcare costs related to diabetes [23, 24]. Research indicates that approximately 25% of DFUs remain unhealed even after one year of treatment, highlighting the chronic and persistent nature of this problem. Alarmingly, more than half of all DFUs are at risk of becoming infected, with about 28% of patients suffering from infected ulcers facing the grim possibility of amputation. This underscores the severe complications and health risks associated with diabetic foot wounds [23, 24]. In summary, the development of (DFUs) is a multifaceted issue exacerbated by sensory loss, delayed treatment, and the body's compromised healing abilities, making prevention and timely management imperative to avoid devastating outcomes.

Although extensive literature exists on diabetic ulcers, most research has predominantly centered on clinical aspects, often overlooking the critical biomechanical factors that contribute to ulcer development. This gap highlights an urgent need for more comprehensive interventions that integrate both prevention and management strategies [25, 26]. Emerging technologies present promising solutions to address this issue. For instance, biomechanics-based prevention strategies that analyze pressure distribution and foot mechanics can help identify at-risk individuals before ulceration occurs. Additionally, smart sensing devices equipped with advanced metrics for real-time monitoring offer the potential for early detection of foot complications, enabling timely intervention. Customized modular insole designs represent another innovative approach, as they can be tailored to the unique biomechanics of each patient's foot. By redistributing pressure more evenly and providing additional support in key areas, these insoles can significantly reduce the risk of ulcer formation [27, 28]. Collectively, these innovations not only hold the promise of enhancing patient care through improved management of foot health but also aim to elevate overall treatment outcomes for individuals living with diabetes [10]. By bridging the existing knowledge gap between clinical practices and biomechanical understanding, we can develop more effective strategies for preventing and managing diabetic ulcers.

1.2 Epidemiology of DFUs

Researchers have found that the prevalence of DFUs is marginally higher in individuals with type 2 diabetes, standing at 6.4%, compared to 5.5% among those with type 1 diabetes. This difference reflects the complex interplay of factors associated with each type of diabetes. Additionally, males are generally at a higher risk of developing DFUs than females, a disparity that can be attributed to various biological and lifestyle factors, including differences in foot care practices, hormonal influences, and underlying health conditions. A particularly striking statistic indicates that one in every six individuals with diabetes is likely to experience a lower limb ulcer at some point in their lives. This highlights the critical importance of early detection and prompt treatment, as studies show that approximately 85% of lower limb amputations are preceded by the presence of an ulcer [10]. Such amputations can drastically impact a patient's quality of life, often leading to mobility issues and necessitating extensive rehabilitation and support services. Moreover, DFUs represent a significant burden on healthcare systems, as they are a leading cause of hospital admissions among diabetic patients, surpassing all other diabetes-related complications in this context. This alarming trend emphasizes the urgent need for effective management strategies to prevent and treat DFUs [29, 30]. Healthcare professionals must prioritize patient education, regular foot examinations, and the implementation of comprehensive care plans to address this serious complication of diabetes. Some key epidemiological insights regarding DFUs include:

- **Prevalence**: DFUs affect an estimated 6.3% of individuals worldwide who are living with diabetes. This condition is notably more common among older adults, as well as those who have been managing diabetes for extended durations. Several factors contribute to the increasing risk of developing DFUs, including poor circulation, which reduces blood flow and hampers the body's ability to heal wounds. Neuropathy, a condition that often arises from prolonged high blood sugar levels, can lead to a loss of sensation in the feet, making individuals unaware of injuries or wounds. Additionally, chronically elevated blood sugar levels can impair the body's natural healing processes, further complicating even minor injuries. These combined factors make DFUs a significant concern in diabetes management, highlighting the need for proactive foot care and regular medical check-ups to prevent complications [3, 13].
- **Ulcer recurrence**: Research shows that nearly 40% of DFUs experience recurrence within just one year after healing, which underscores the critical challenges faced in the management of these wounds. Moreover, the recurrence rate escalates dramatically, with approximately 65% of DFUs reappearing within five years. These alarming statistics not only highlight the complexities in treating DFUs but also emphasize the urgent necessity for comprehensive, long-term preventive strategies. Effective management must focus not only on immediate healing but also on addressing the underlying risk factors and implementing proactive measures to reduce the likelihood of recurrence, ultimately aiming to improve the overall quality of life for individuals affected by this condition.
- **Amputation risk**: DFUs represent a serious complication for individuals with diabetes, with a concerning 14% to 24% of these cases ultimately leading to lower limb amputation. This statistic highlights the urgent need for proactive measures in preventing DFUs, which is essential for comprehensive diabetes management. Effective prevention strategies involve a multifaceted approach that includes prioritizing foot care through regular examinations and proper hygiene practices. Patients should be educated on the importance of daily foot inspections to identify early signs of ulceration, such as redness, swelling, or any breaks in the skin. Additionally, appropriate footwear is crucial to prevent injuries that could exacerbate the risk. Healthcare providers play a vital role by implementing regular foot assessments as part of routine diabetic care and ensuring timely intervention when issues arise. Encouraging patients to actively participate in their care, by maintaining optimal blood glucose levels and adhering to treatment plans, can further mitigate the risk of developing DFUs [13, 27]. By fostering awareness

and promoting effective strategies, we can significantly decrease the incidence of DFUs and their associated complications, ultimately improving the quality of life for those living with diabetes.

- **Economic burden**: The financial implications of treating DFUs are extensive and multifaceted, encompassing a wide array of expenses that significantly burden both patients and healthcare systems. Key components of these costs include hospitalizations, surgical procedures, and ongoing wound care management. Hospitalizations can often be necessary for intravenous antibiotic therapy or to address acute complications such as infections. Each hospital visit adds to the cumulative financial toll, particularly if patients experience recurrent episodes that require additional treatments. Surgical interventions, too, represent a significant cost factor. Patients may undergo procedures to remove necrotic tissue or more advanced surgeries such as limb salvage operations, each of which incurs substantial expenses for both the procedure itself and postoperative care. The chronicity of DFUs complicates their management further, as patients typically require long-term care plans. This can encompass a variety of specialized dressings that promote healing and prevent infections, which can be more expensive than standard wound care supplies. Regular monitoring by healthcare professionals is also essential, often involving consistent follow-up appointments that can add to the financial strain faced by patients. Additionally, successful management of DFUs frequently necessitates a multidisciplinary approach, involving collaboration between podiatrists, wound care specialists, endocrinologists, and primary care providers. This teamwork, while beneficial for patient outcomes, can lead to higher overall costs due to the need for coordinated efforts across multiple healthcare disciplines. As these expenses accumulate, they place a significant strain on healthcare systems worldwide. Resources that could be allocated to other critical areas of patient care are diverted to manage the complications arising from DFUs, highlighting the need for effective prevention and management strategies to mitigate not only the financial burden but also the impact on patient quality of life.

India serves as a poignant illustration of the escalating global diabetes epidemic, where a complex interplay of socioeconomic factors, cultural practices, and inadequate access to high-quality diabetic foot care exacerbates the issue of diabetic foot ulceration. With an alarming estimate of 62 million individuals diagnosed with diabetes, the prevalence of DFUs is steadily increasing, posing significant health challenges. Approximately 50% of those suffering from DFUs develop infections, and among this subset, nearly 20% may face the distressing prospect of amputation. The gravity of this situation is underscored by alarming statistics: DFUs account for roughly 80% of all nontraumatic lower-limb amputations in India each year. In urban settings, research has revealed that around 15.3% of diabetic patients with foot complications ultimately undergo either major or minor amputations 33. These figures highlight a crucial public health concern that calls for urgent action. The need for enhanced diabetic foot care services is paramount. This involves not only improving healthcare infrastructures but also implementing comprehensive public awareness campaigns aimed at educating patients and healthcare providers about the risks associated with DFUs and the importance of early intervention. Greater accessibility to healthcare resources, especially for marginalized and vulnerable communities, is essential to address these pressing issues effectively. By prioritizing these areas, we have the potential to significantly reduce the incidence of diabetes-related complications and enhance the quality of life for millions living with this chronic condition in India. It is imperative that we tackle these challenges with urgency and dedication to prevent unnecessary suffering and improve health outcomes across the population [32].

The increasing prevalence of diabetes in India, coupled with its associated complications, has significantly expanded the ulceration treatment market in the country. As of 2023, this market was valued at USD 213.7 million and is projected to experience a robust compound annual growth rate (CAGR) of 7.82% from 2024 to 2030. Several critical factors underpin this notable growth. Firstly, the rising incidence of diabetes among the Indian population is alarmingly high. An estimated 77 million people in India are living with diabetes, a number expected to rise due to lifestyle factors such as unhealthy diets, sedentary behavior, and urbanization 13. Poorly managed blood glucose levels increase the risk of developing DFUs, which can lead to severe complications such as infections or even amputations if left untreated. Moreover, the aging population in India plays a significant role in this dynamic. As the demographic shift towards an older population continues, a greater number of individuals are experiencing chronic health conditions, including various forms of diabetes. Older adults are particularly vulnerable not only due to the physiological changes that accompany aging but also because they often manage multiple health issues concurrently, which can complicate diabetes management and increase the risk of foot complications. The challenge of DFUs represents a considerable global health crisis, with India bearing a substantial proportion of this burden. According to medical studies, up to 25% of diabetes patients will develop foot ulcers in their lifetime, highlighting the urgency for effective intervention strategies [2, 3, 27]. The high prevalence of diabetes and its associated complications underscores the need for comprehensive approaches that include not only prevention and early detection but also effective management of DFUs. To mitigate the impact of DFUs on both individuals and healthcare systems, stakeholders must prioritize awareness campaigns, patient education, and access to advanced medical treatments. These strategies are essential for improving outcomes and reducing healthcare costs associated with diabetes-related complications. Addressing the DFU challenge in India requires a multifaceted approach that leverages technological innovations, healthcare infrastructures, and community support systems, ultimately striving for a healthier future for millions at risk.

1.3 Importance of Biomechanics in Diabetic Foot Ulceration

Biomechanical factors are instrumental in the development and progression of DFUs. Several key contributors to ulcer formation include the irregular distribution of plantar pressure, altered gait patterns, and increased tissue stiffness, all of which can exert excessive stress on specific areas of the foot. These pressures create conditions that are conducive to ulceration, especially in individuals with underlying conditions such as diabetes, which may compromise their healing ability. To thoroughly understand and address these biomechanical issues, researchers and clinicians utilize advanced finite element models [33–37]. These simulations replicate the complex biomechanical stresses the foot endures during various physical activities, such as walking, running, and standing. By analyzing these models, they can pinpoint specific areas at high risk for ulceration, thereby facilitating the design of targeted intervention strategies aimed at minimizing these risks. One significant intervention being explored is the design of advanced smart pressure-sensing insoles. These innovative devices are equipped with sensors that provide real-time feedback on pressure distribution across the foot, allowing users to adjust their movements and posture to prevent excessive stress on vulnerable areas (see Fig. 1.1). Furthermore, the development of customized 3D-printed modular insoles is gaining traction. These insoles can be tailored to conform to an individual's unique foot structure and biomechanics, offering optimal support and effective pressure redistribution. The primary objective of these interventions is to redistribute plantar pressure and significantly reduce the risk of ulceration. Achieving this can have profound implications, as it not only helps to prevent DFUs but also mitigates the risk of severe complications, including infections and amputations, which can be life-altering for many individuals.

The incidence of DFUs is closely linked to a variety of biomechanical abnormalities in the foot, which can typically be classified into several categories. These include abnormal arch structure, wherein an excessively high or low arch can affect weight

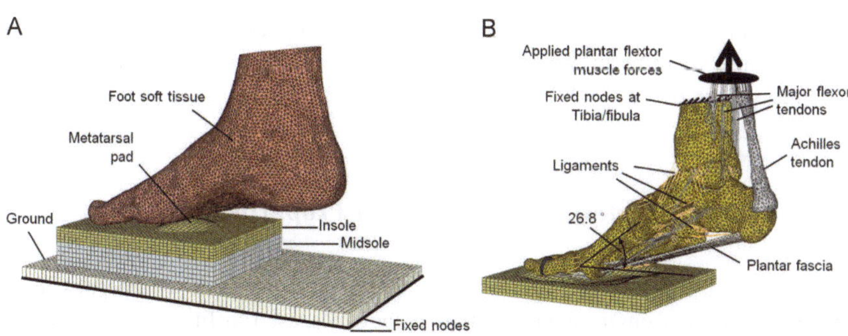

Fig. 1.1 **a** Finite element models of the human foot, and the supporting surface consisting of metatarsal pad, insole, and midsole, and **b** The applied loading and boundary conditions to simulate a muscle-demanding instant in gait. *Reproduced with permission from IOP Science* 13

distribution; excessive joint motion, which can lead to instability and abnormal stress on soft tissues; and neuropathy-related variations in sensory feedback, which hinder the individual's ability to perceive pain or discomfort resulting from pressure buildup. A comprehensive understanding of these categories is crucial for developing effective preventive strategies and treatment protocols tailored to individuals at risk for DFUs. By addressing the underlying biomechanical factors, healthcare professionals can implement more effective management strategies to enhance foot health and ensure better quality of life for those affected.

1.3.1 Plantar Pressure Distribution

Individuals with diabetes often experience high plantar pressure at specific locations on the foot, particularly the metatarsal heads, heel, and toes. These areas are prone to developing ulcers due to the excess pressure, which can cause significant damage to both the skin and underlying tissues. The resulting tissue breakdown can lead to ischemia, a condition where there is insufficient blood flow, further exacerbating the risk of ulceration and complications. Understanding the patterns of plantar pressure is crucial for creating effective offloading interventions designed to redistribute this pressure away from vulnerable sites. By analyzing gait mechanics and using pressure mapping, healthcare professionals can identify high-pressure zones with greater precision. To mitigate the risk of ulcer formation, a variety of strategies can be employed. Custom orthotics are designed to accommodate the unique contours of an individual's foot and redistribute pressure more evenly. Specialized footwear can provide additional support and cushioning, further alleviating stress on susceptible areas. Pressure relief techniques, such as using foam inserts or adjusting walking habits, can also contribute significantly to foot health [3, 38]. Additionally, early identification and proactive management of high-pressure zones are vital in preventing severe complications. By addressing these risks promptly, healthcare providers can significantly lower the likelihood of severe infections and amputations, ultimately enhancing the quality of life for individuals living with diabetes. By prioritizing foot care and implementing preventive measures, we can foster better health outcomes and improve the overall well-being of this population.

1.3.2 Tissue Stiffness and Mechanical Properties

Diabetic foot tissues undergo significant changes in their mechanical properties due to altered biochemical environments, which include increased stiffness, decreased elasticity, and reduced tensile strength. These changes in tissue composition result from factors such as chronic hyperglycemia, neuropathy, and poor circulation, commonly associated with diabetes. Consequently, these tissues become more susceptible to damage, particularly during repetitive loading activities like walking or standing for prolonged periods. As a result, individuals with diabetes face an elevated risk of developing foot ulcers, which can lead to severe complications such as infections or even amputations if left untreated. These ulcers often arise unnoticed due to peripheral neuropathy, which diminishes sensation in the feet, making it difficult for individuals to detect injuries or pressure sores before they worsen. To better understand the risks associated with DFUs, researchers employ finite element modeling (FEM), a sophisticated simulation technique that allows for a comprehensive analysis of the mechanical behavior of diabetic foot tissues [11, 13]. By modeling the response of these tissues to varying mechanical stresses, FEM provides valuable insights into the specific conditions that contribute to ulcer formation. This research is essential for developing targeted preventive strategies and therapies to enhance foot health in individuals with diabetes, ultimately reducing the incidence of foot-related complications.

1.3.3 Gait and Postural Alterations

Diabetic neuropathy profoundly impacts motor control and presents a variety of challenges, particularly in the context of gait and mobility. Individuals with this condition may experience an unsteady gait characterized by inconsistent step length and altered foot positioning, which increases the pressure on specific areas of the foot, such as the heels and balls. This mechanical stress is a significant factor that escalates the risk of developing foot ulcers, a prevalent and serious complication for those with diabetes. The intricate relationship between these gait changes and foot health necessitates a thorough understanding for effective prevention and treatment strategies. Researchers are now leveraging advanced computational modeling techniques to precisely simulate the gait patterns associated with diabetes. This sophisticated approach allows for a detailed examination of the underlying biomechanics, revealing critical insights into how diabetic neuropathy alters movement and increases injury risk. With this knowledge, healthcare professionals can design personalized orthotic solutions that are specifically tailored to the unique needs of each patient [11, 13]. These customized devices aim to distribute pressure more evenly across the foot, enhance stability during movement, and ultimately promote safer ambulation. By addressing the intricacies of diabetic gait, these interventions not only improve mobility but also significantly reduce the likelihood of ulceration, thereby enhancing the overall quality of life for individuals living with diabetes.

1.3.4 Offloading Strategies and Interventions

A variety of offloading techniques, which include total contact casting, therapeutic footwear, and a range of specialized insoles, have been widely employed to prevent DFUs, a common and serious complication for individuals living with diabetes. While these standardized interventions are designed to reduce pressure on vulnerable areas of the foot, they often fall short in providing sufficient protection. This shortcoming arises from their failure to consider the unique anatomical and biomechanical variations that exist in each patient's foot. These individual differences can significantly alter the distribution of pressure during activities such as walking and standing, ultimately influencing the overall effectiveness of offloading methods. In response to these challenges, this study seeks to explore the development of customized insole designs that are specifically tailored to each patient's distinct foot structure and movement patterns. The approach emphasizes the importance of personalization in addressing the complex interactions between foot anatomy and pressure distribution [12, 28]. Additionally, the study integrates an innovative method of real-time pressure monitoring, which facilitates immediate feedback on pressure distribution across the foot. This dual strategy, combining personalized insoles with advanced monitoring technology, aims to enhance the efficacy of offloading strategies. The ultimate goal is to significantly reduce the incidence of DFUs and improve overall patient outcomes, making strides towards better management of diabetic foot complications [27].

1.4 Computational Modeling of Diabetic Foot and Ulcers

In the area of biomechanical research, while traditional experimental analyses have often concentrated on assessing interfacial variables such as pressure distributions at tissue interfaces, the development of reliable numerical models can significantly enhance our understanding. These models not only illuminate interfacial pressures but also delve into the internal stresses and strains experienced by plantar tissues under a variety of physiological and mechanical conditions 41. FEMs have gained widespread acceptance in biomechanical studies due to their exceptional capability to accurately represent anatomical structures characterized by irregular geometries and complex material behaviors. These sophisticated models simulate challenging boundary conditions and varying loading scenarios, enabling researchers to perform both static and dynamic analyses with remarkable precision and efficiency (see Fig. 1.2). The versatility of FEMs allows for the exploration of different foot postures, gait patterns, and even the influence of footwear on tissue response [40]. In recent years, computational modeling and simulation have emerged as indispensable tools in the examination of diabetic foot biomechanics. Their application is particularly critical in developing targeted interventions aimed at preventing DFUs, which pose a significant risk for individuals suffering from diabetes. Prior research has meticulously analyzed various factors, such as the size and anatomical location of ulcers, and their correlation with plantar pressures, thus providing insightful revelations into the mechanisms that drive ulcer progression and severity [41]. Despite the promising advancements in this field, a comprehensive understanding of the complex interactions between biomechanical factors, the mechanical properties of various soft tissues, and the effects of different therapeutic interventions on ulcer healing and prevention continues to be a dynamic area of active investigation. This ongoing

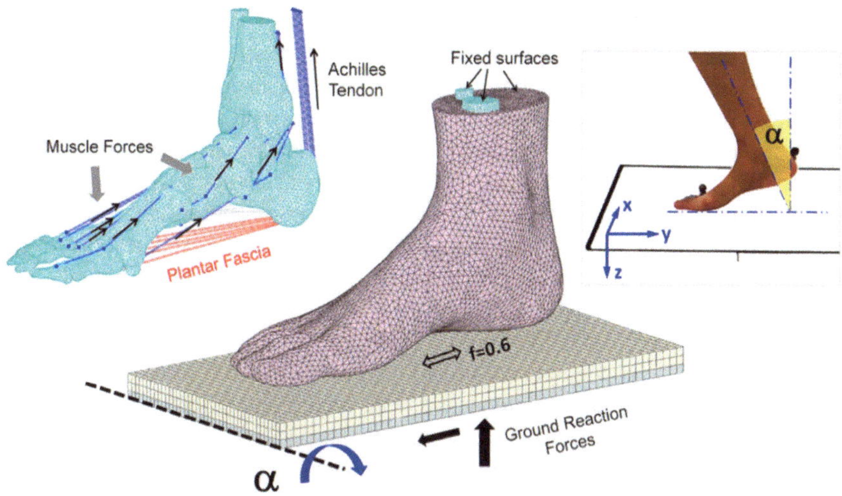

Fig. 1.2 The three-dimensional finite element model of the foot and ankle and application of boundary and loading conditions. *Reproduced with permission from IOP Science* 13

research is crucial for developing effective treatment strategies that can enhance patient outcomes and minimize complications related to foot ulcers. By interweaving principles of biomechanics, material science, and clinical practice, we can develop a holistic approach to patient care that is tailored to the unique needs of individuals at risk for foot ulcers.

1.5 Intervention Development for DFUs

The management of DFUs presents a multifaceted and persistent challenge in the field of medicine, despite the wide range of advanced medical and surgical interventions currently available. These ulcers are not only common but also notoriously prone to recurrence; alarming statistics indicate that up to 85% of lower-limb amputations in diabetic patients are preceded by the onset of a foot ulcer. Such scenarios highlight the urgent necessity for effective prevention and management strategies that can mitigate the risks associated with DFUs. To tackle the complexities surrounding DFUs, various innovative and evidence-based approaches can be deployed. Among these are customized footwear and unloading orthoses, as well as advanced therapeutic strategies. These interventions are specifically designed to redistribute plantar pressures across the foot, which can significantly alleviate the mechanical stress on ulcer-affected areas. By effectively reducing the pressure exerted on the plantar surface, orthotic devices not only relieve tension in ulcerated sites but also create an optimal environment for healing. The primary objective of these medical interventions is to reallocate the pressure that the plantar fascia, a crucial structure that supports the foot, experiences. When subjected to excessive stress, the plantar fascia can contribute to ulcer formation, making its protection vital.

To effectively customize foot orthoses, practitioners can utilize a diverse range of materials, each varying in density, cushioning properties, and shock absorption capabilities. This allows for a highly personalized treatment approach that can be tailored to meet the specific needs of each patient, enhancing both comfort and efficacy. While numerous unloading modalities exist, selecting the most appropriate technique is influenced by multiple factors, including the specific location and severity of the ulcer, the patient's unique physical characteristics, and their ability to comply with the prescribed treatment regimen. Among the available options, total contact casts (TCCs) have been recognized as the most effective offloading method for managing neuropathic DFUs, as documented in various studies [42, 43]. Total contact casts are uniquely designed to accommodate a heel, facilitating ambulation while safeguarding the ulcerated area. They are accurately shaped to conform to the contours of the patient's foot, utilizing minimal padding to ensure effective pressure distribution. The primary purpose of TCCs is to provide protective coverage to the ulcer while evenly distributing pressure across the entire surface of the foot. This method not only alleviates pressure from the ulcer itself but also fosters a healing-friendly environment, ultimately promoting recovery and reducing the risk of complications (see Fig. 1.3). Overall, a comprehensive understanding of these innovative strategies and proper implementation can greatly enhance the management of DFUs, significantly improving patient outcomes and reducing the incidence of limb amputations.

To effectively manage and alleviate forefoot or midfoot ulcers, the utilization of nonremovable TCCs is highly recommended. These specialized casts are significantly designed to allow for limited weight-bearing activity while ensuring complete immobilization of the affected foot, thereby fostering optimal conditions for healing [45]. One of the significant advantages of TCCs is their inherent feature of being nonremovable by patients themselves. This restriction greatly enhances compliance with treatment protocols, as patients are less likely to inadvertently remove the cast,

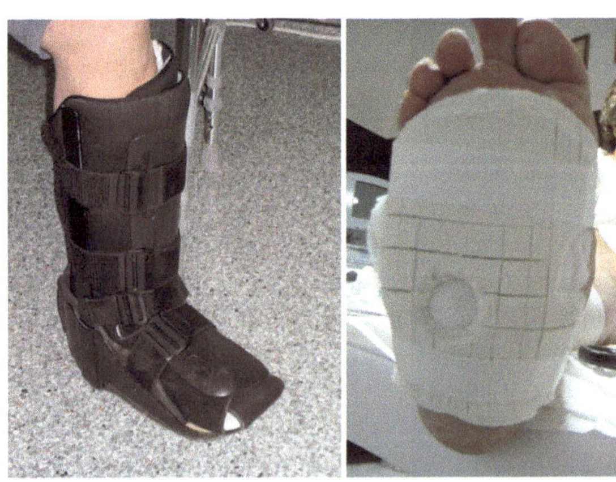

(A) (B)

Fig. 1.3 **a** Removable cast walker and **b** Offloading of a diabetic foot ulcer with felted foam. *Reproduced under the terms of the Creative Commons Attribution 2.0 International License* 46 which could undermine the healing process. The enforced immobilization associated with TCCs leads to decreased activity levels, contributing to a more effective wound healing process by reducing mechanical stress on the ulcerated area [46]. However, despite their benefits, TCCs present challenges that need to be addressed for successful implementation. One of the primary concerns is the necessity for skilled application by trained healthcare professionals. Many healthcare facilities, particularly those in community settings, often face a shortage of personnel with specialized training, such as podiatrists or certified cast technicians, who have the expertise required to apply these casts correctly. Improper application of a TCC can result in various complications, including skin irritation, pressure sores, and, in rare instances, exacerbation of the ulcers being treated. This reality underscores the critical importance of comprehensive training in the application of TCCs to prevent adverse outcomes and ensure safe patient management [38, 47–49]. In contrast to prefabricated orthoses, which may not always provide the necessary support, customized foot orthoses offer a more tailored approach to treatment. These orthoses are specifically designed to achieve complete and precise contact with the plantar surface of the foot, maximizing support and effectively offloading the regions most affected by ulcers [50, 51]. Despite the advantages of customized orthoses, there are still limitations to their overall effectiveness. This limitation highlights the pioneering need for the development of more innovative and personalized therapeutic solutions that can address the unique needs of each patient, ultimately enhancing healing outcomes and improving quality of life for individuals suffering from foot ulcers.

1.6 Research Gap

Current research on the biomechanics of the diabetic foot is severely limited, hindering our understanding of how foot ulcers develop and progress. A comprehensive examination of the mechanical forces and interactions at play is crucial for identifying the precise factors that contribute to ulcer formation in diabetic patients. Moreover, there is a significant gap in knowledge regarding effective strategies for preventing diabetic ulceration. Understanding the underlying mechanisms that lead to skin breakdown in vulnerable individuals can help develop targeted interventions and education to mitigate risks. Additionally, the field lacks an effective, patient-specific pressure offloading device tailored to address ulceration risks at various sites on the foot. The development of such a customized offloading solution is essential in preventing ulcers by ensuring that pressure distribution is optimized for each individual's unique anatomical and physiological needs. Through such advancements, we can enhance care for those at risk of diabetic foot complications.

Due to the limitations in current literature, there is a pressing need for patient-specific biomechanical solutions. This includes the development of computational modeling, smart pressure monitoring systems, and modular insole designs. The findings from this work are expected to make a substantial contribution to our understanding of diabetic foot ulceration and the strategies for its prevention. This work highlights the integration of advanced computational modeling techniques, the development of innovative medical devices, and their clinical significance, thereby illustrating the potential for translating these advancements into practical solutions that can alleviate the burden of DFUs. A key innovation arising from this study is the novel modular insole, designed specifically for individual patients. This customized offloading insole aims to significantly enhance the quality of life for those afflicted by diabetic ulcers. By strategically redistributing pressure away from the plantar area of the foot, the insole not only reduces pain but also promotes better mobility. The personalized nature of the insole ensures that it meets the unique needs of each patient, thereby offering a tailored approach to treatment that could play a pivotal role in preventing ulceration and supporting the overall well-being of individuals living with diabetes.

References

1. Sun H et al (2022) IDF Diabetes Atlas: Global, regional and country-level diabetes prevalence estimates for 2021 and projections for 2045. Diabetes Res Clin Pract 183:109119
2. Gupta S et al (2023) Diabot: development of a diabetic foot pressure tracking device. J 6, 32–47
3. Bose D, Singh G, Gupta S, Chanda A (2024) Development of a Novel Customized Insole for Effective Pressure Offloading in Diabetic Patients. Prosthesis 6:341–356
4. Wu HJ et al (2022) The promising hydrogel candidates for preclinically treating diabetic foot ulcer: a systematic review and meta-analysis. Adv Wound Care 12:28–37
5. Rai V, Moellmer R, Agrawal DK (2022) Clinically relevant experimental rodent models of diabetic foot ulcer. Mol Cell Biochem 477:1239–1247
6. Bakker K, Abbas Z, Pendsey S (2006) Step by Step, improving diabetic foot care in the developing world. Pract Diabetes Int. 23:365–369
7. Moulik PK, Mtonga R, Gill GV (2003) Amputation and mortality in new-onset diabetic foot ulcers stratified by etiology. Diabetes Care 26:491–494
8. Mishra SC, Chhatbar KC, Kashikar A, Mehndiratta A (2017) Diabetic foot. BMJ 359:j5064
9. Armstrong DG, Boulton AJM, Bus SA (2017) Diabetic foot ulcers and their recurrence. N Engl J Med 376:2367–2375
10. Zhang P et al (2017) Global epidemiology of diabetic foot ulceration: a systematic review and meta-analysis†. Ann Med 49:106–116
11. Singh G, Lamba A, Chanda A (2024) Role of additive manufacturing for the management of diabetic foot ulcers. In Addit Manuf Biomed Appl 19–38 (Springer, Singapore). https://doi.org/10.1007/978-981-97-5456-4_2
12. Fernando ME et al (2016) Plantar pressures are higher in cases with diabetic foot ulcers compared to controls despite a longer stance phase duration. BMC Endocr Disord 16:51
13. Singh G, Chanda A (2024) Finite element modeling of diabetic foot: a state-of-the-art review. Eng Res Express 6:012507
14. Amin N, Doupis J (2016) Diabetic foot disease: From the evaluation of the "foot at risk" to the novel diabetic ulcer treatment modalities. World J Diabetes 7:153
15. Naves CCLM (2016) The diabetic foot: a historical overview and gaps in current treatment. Adv Wound Care 5:191–197
16. Pecoraro RE, Reiber GE, Burgess EM (1990) Pathways to diabetic limb amputation: Basis for prevention. Diabetes Care 13:513–521
17. Cavanagh PR, Lipsky BA, Bradbury AW, Botek G (2005) Treatment for diabetic foot ulcers. Lancet 366:1725–1735

18. Aumiller WD, Dollahite HA (2015) Pathogenesis and management of diabetic foot ulcers. J Am Acad Physician Assist. 28:28–34
19. Boulton AJM (2008) The diabetic foot: grand overview, epidemiology and pathogenesis. Diabetes Metab Res Rev 24:S3–S6
20. Prompers L et al (2008) Resource utilisation and costs associated with the treatment of diabetic foot ulcers. Prospective data from the eurodiale study. Diabetologia 51, 1826–1834
21. Prompers L et al (2007) High prevalence of ischaemia, infection and serious comorbidity in patients with diabetic foot disease in Europe. Baseline results from the Eurodiale study. Diabetologia 50, 18–25
22. Selth CA, Francis BE (2000) Review of non-functional plantar heel pain. Foot 10 97–104 at https://doi.org/10.1054/foot.2000.0609
23. Driver VR, Fabbi M, Lavery LA, Gibbons G (2010) The costs of diabetic foot: The economic case for the limb salvage team. J Vasc Surg 52:17S-22S
24. Prompers L et al (2008) Prediction of outcome in individuals with diabetic foot ulcers: Focus on the differences between individuals with and without peripheral arterial disease. The EURODIALE Study. Diabetologia 51:747–755
25. Pickwell K et al (2015) Predictors of lower-extremity amputation in patients with an infected diabetic foot ulcer. Diabetes Care 38:852–857
26. Voelker R (2023) What are diabetic foot ulcers? JAMA 330:2314–2314
27. Singh G, Bose D, Chanda A (2025) Development and testing of a novel diabetic orthosis for plantar pressure reduction. Facta Univ Ser Mech Eng. https://doi.org/10.22190/FUME240725044S
28. Owings TM et al (2009) Plantar pressures in diabetic patients with foot ulcers which have remained healed. Diabet Med 26:1141–1146
29. Gupta S, Singh G, Chanda A (2021) Prediction of diabetic foot ulcer progression: a computational study. Biomed Phys Eng Express 7:065020
30. Singh G, Gupta S, Chanda A (2021) Biomechanical modelling of diabetic foot ulcers: A computational study. J Biomech 127:110699
31. Ghosh P, Valia R (2017) Burden of diabetic foot ulcers in india: evidence landscape from published literature. Value Heal. 20:A485
32. Patil P et al (2023) The burden of diabetic foot ulcers in urban India. Indian J Endocrinol Metab. https://doi.org/10.4103/IJEM.IJEM_346_22
33. Singh G, Chanda A (2022) Biomechanical modeling of progressive wound healing: A computational study. Biomed Eng Adv. 4:100055
34. Finite A, Gupta V, Chanda A (2023) Finite element analysis of hierarchical metamaterial-based patterns for generating high expansion in skin grafting. Math Comput Appl, 28, Page 89
35. Gupta V, Garg A, Tewari N, Srivastav S, Chanda A (2024) Development of patient-specific finite element model for study of composite dental implants. Biomed Phys Eng Express 10:025035
36. Chanda A, Unnikrishnan V, Roy S, Richter HE (2015) Computational modeling of the female pelvic support structures and organs to understand the mechanism of pelvic organ prolapse: a review. Appl Mech Rev 67 at https://doi.org/10.1115/1.4030967
37. Chanda A, Upchurch W (2018) Biomechanical modeling of wounded skin. J Compos Sci, 2, 69 2, 69
38. Chhikara K, Singh G, Gupta S, Chanda A (2022) Progress of additive manufacturing in fabrication of foot orthoses for diabetic patients: A review. Ann 3D Print Med 8, 100085
39. Yarnitzky G, Yizhar Z, Gefen A (2006) Real-time subject-specific monitoring of internal deformations and stresses in the soft tissues of the foot: A new approach in gait analysis. J Biomech 39:2673–2689
40. Guiotto A, Sawacha Z, Guarneri G, Avogaro A, Cobelli C (2014) 3D finite element model of the diabetic neuropathic foot: A gait analysis driven approach. J Biomech 47:3064–3071
41. Yadav AK et al (2023) Comparative study of various dressing techniques in diabetic foot ulcers in the Indian population: a single-center experience. Int J Diabetes Dev Ctries. 43:647–653
42. Armstrong DG, Lavery LA, Nixon BP, Boulton AJM (2004) It's not what you put on, but what you take off: techniques for debriding and off-loading the diabetic foot wound. Clin Infect Dis 39:S92–S99

43. Rathur HM, Boulton AJM (2007) The diabetic foot. Clin Dermatol 25:109–120
44. Alexiadou K, Doupis J (2012) Management of diabetic foot ulcers. Diabetes Ther. 3:1–15
45. Burns J, Begg L (2011) Optimizing the offloading properties of the total contact cast for plantar foot ulceration. Diabet Med 28:179–185
46. Boulton AJM (2004) Pressure and the diabetic foot: clinical science and offloading techniques. Am J Surg 187:S17–S24
47. Whiting DR, Guariguata L, Weil C, Shaw J (2011) IDF Diabetes Atlas: Global estimates of the prevalence of diabetes for 2011 and 2030. Diabetes Res Clin Pract 94:311–321
48. Katsilambros N, Dounis E, Makrilakis K, Tentolouris N, Tsapogas P (2011) Atlas of the Diabetic Foot. Atlas Diabet. Foot 1–249 https://doi.org/10.1002/9781444317589
49. Aalaa M, Malazy OT, Sanjari M, Peimani M, Mohajeri-Tehrani MR (2012) Nurses' role in diabetic foot prevention and care; a review. J Diabetes Metab Disord 11:1–6
50. Chanda A, Unnikrishnan V (2018) Novel insole design for diabetic foot ulcer management. Proc Inst Mech Eng Part H J Eng Med 232, 1182–1195
51. Dubský M et al (2013) Risk factors for recurrence of diabetic foot ulcers: prospective follow-up analysis in the Eurodiale subgroup. Int Wound J 10:555–561

Chapter 2
Literature on Finite Element Modeling

2.1 Introduction

Diabetic foot ulcers (DFUs) are a significant healthcare challenge that greatly impacts the quality of life for individuals living with diabetes. These ulcers often result from a combination of factors, including neuropathy, peripheral artery disease, and impaired wound healing, all of which can lead to severe consequences such as infections, amputations, and increased healthcare costs. To effectively address this issue, it is crucial to understand the underlying biomechanical factors that contribute to the formation and progression of these ulcers. One of the most promising research tools in this field is finite element analysis (FEA). FEA allows researchers to create detailed, computer-generated models that simulate the complex biomechanics of the diabetic foot [1, 2]. This innovative approach enables the investigation of how various anatomical structures, such as bones, soft tissues, and blood vessels, respond to different mechanical loads and conditions encountered during daily activities. Importantly, FEA facilitates the examination of critical biomechanical factors that contribute to ulcer development. For instance, it can be used to analyze pressure distribution across the foot, identify areas of high shear forces that may lead to tissue breakdown, and assess how tissue deformation occurs under specific conditions. By gaining insights into these mechanisms, researchers can better understand how foot ulcers initiate and progress, leading to more targeted prevention and treatment strategies [3, 4].

This chapter aims to provide an in-depth overview of the current research landscape surrounding DFUs and finite element modeling (FEM). It will highlight key findings from recent studies, showcasing how FEA has advanced our understanding of the biomechanical environment surrounding diabetic foot. Additionally, the review will discuss the implications of these findings for clinical practice, particularly in terms of developing more effective preventative measures and treatment protocols. Furthermore, the review will explore the potential applications of interventions that leverage insights gained from FEM, such as custom orthotics, footwear modifications, and therapeutic approaches that enhance circulation and healing. By integrating

A. Chanda and G. Singh, *Diabetic Foot Ulcer*, Biomedical Materials for Multi-functional Applications, https://doi.org/10.1007/978-981-95-2484-6_2

these strategies, healthcare providers can significantly improve patient outcomes, reduce the incidence and severity of DFUs, and ultimately lower the burden of healthcare costs associated with these serious complications.

The human foot is a remarkably complex anatomical structure composed of over 26 bones, numerous joints, a network of ligaments, tendons, and various soft tissues. Each component plays a crucial role in facilitating movement and ensuring stability during various activities such as walking, running, and jumping [5]. This intricate design is essential for mobility; however, it also presents significant challenges for researchers who seek to conduct in vivo measurements [6, 7]. Understanding the physiological stresses and strains the foot encounters under functional loading conditions can be difficult due to the foot's complexity and the dynamic nature of its biomechanics. To navigate these challenges, researchers have increasingly adopted advanced computer-based simulations, particularly FEA, as a means to accurately replicate the biomechanical behavior of the foot [8, 9]. These simulation methods enable detailed modeling of the foot's complex structure and interactions under a variety of conditions. This approach has gained significant recognition for its effectiveness in assessing not just general foot mechanics but also specific conditions such as diabetic foot complications. One of the primary advantages of utilizing FEA in the study of foot mechanics is its capacity for parametric investigations. This allows researchers to systematically modify various variables, such as load distributions, material properties, and anatomical configurations, to observe their effects on foot behavior [10]. As a result, researchers can gain profound insights into the physiological functioning and progression of conditions like DFUs. FEA facilitates a thorough evaluation of the mechanical responses of diverse biological tissues in the foot, including the skin's tensile properties, the cushioning effects of fat pads, the flexibility of tendons, and the strength and stability provided by ligaments [11]. The precision and level of detail offered by FEA make it an invaluable tool in biomechanical research. It provides insights that may be unattainable through traditional in vivo or cadaveric testing, which often involve ethical considerations, logistical challenges, and are resource intensive. By employing FEA, researchers can derive a holistic understanding of the underlying mechanics influencing foot health, thereby contributing to improved clinical outcomes for patients with diabetes and enhancing treatment protocols. Despite the numerous benefits that FEA offers, there remains a conspicuous gap in the literature concerning the application of computational modeling in the examination of foot biomechanics, particularly in the context of diabetic ulceration [12–15]. While many studies have investigated various anatomical components of the human body, comprehensive research focused on leveraging computational methods to explore diabetic foot ulceration is still limited. Addressing this gap could pave the way for pioneering approaches to prevent and manage diabetic foot complications, ultimately improving patient care and outcomes in this critical area of healthcare.

2.2 Foot Modeling

The foot, as the lowest part of the body, plays a critical role in supporting weight and facilitating movement, enduring substantial forces that fluctuate widely depending on the type of activity being performed, whether walking, running, or standing. Despite its vital importance to mobility and overall balance, modeling the foot accurately remains a challenging task due to several factors, including its complex anatomical structure, considerable individual variations, and the dynamic nature of foot movement [16, 17]. Advancements in biomechanics and 3D modeling technologies are essential for deepening our understanding of foot function. This knowledge is pivotal not only for enhancing footwear design but also for developing effective orthotics and treatments for various foot-related conditions, such as DFUs. These ulcers arise due to a combination of factors, including neuropathy and poor circulation, making accurate foot modeling particularly significant for preventative care and management. The FEA technique stands out as a crucial tool in this area, allowing researchers to investigate mechanical interactions at both macroscopic levels, such as the overall structure of the foot, and microscopic levels, which include the behavior of individual cells and tissues under stress. Several finite element software packages exist, each tailored with unique features and limitations. Among the most prominent are Ansys and LS-Dyna, both renowned for their advanced simulation capabilities, which enable detailed modeling of complex mechanical interactions not just within the foot but across a range of biological systems. The development of an accurate foot model is a multistep process that begins with a thorough definition of the foot's anatomical structures [6, 7]. This includes detailed representations of bones, ligaments, tendons, and soft tissues. For instance, two-dimensional models, often utilized in research focusing on DFUs, typically rely on cross-sectional views that concentrate on either the sagittal or coronal plane. This method simplifies the modeling workflow and speeds up solution times when compared to more complex three-dimensional models. However, it is important to acknowledge the inherent limitations of two-dimensional models. While they facilitate quicker analysis and can be effective for certain types of studies, they may fail to capture the full complexity of tissue deformations that occur in three dimensions, especially those that happen outside the observable plane [18, 19]. This shortcoming emphasizes the necessity for further advancements in modeling techniques that not only enhance accuracy but also enrich our insights into the intricate biological systems involved in foot mechanics and health. Developing more sophisticated models will ultimately contribute to better diagnoses, tailored treatments, and improved outcomes for individuals with foot-related ailments.

To address the inherent limitations of traditional modeling techniques, researchers have increasingly turned to advanced imaging modalities, including X-rays, computed tomography (CT), and magnetic resonance imaging (MRI). These sophisticated technologies allow for the creation of highly customized and detailed anatomical foot models, as illustrated in Fig. 2.1 [20–22]. These imaging methods provide intricate insights into the complex structural composition of the foot, capturing its

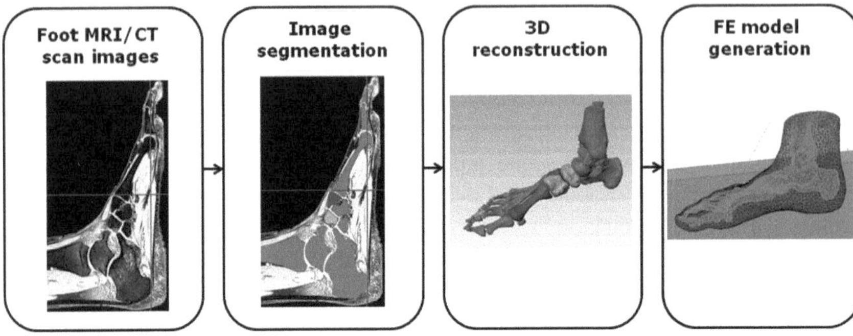

Fig. 2.1 Workflow of the development of the FE foot model. *Reproduced with permission from IOP Science* [1]

nuanced features such as bone density, soft tissue composition, and vascular structures. This level of detail is critical for developing models that truly reflect real human anatomy, thereby enhancing our understanding of various conditions affecting the foot. For the accurate representation of anatomical features in three-dimensional modeling, researchers have employed advanced image segmentation techniques. These techniques enable the visualization of progressive changes in diabetic foot conditions, facilitating early diagnosis and more effective treatment plans [23, 24]. Despite their advantages, these imaging techniques are not without drawbacks. They tend to be both expensive and time-consuming, often requiring specialized equipment and expertise. Furthermore, many of these methods depend on anatomical images derived from dissected cadavers, which may pose ethical concerns and are not always readily available, thereby limiting accessibility for widespread research and application. This highlights the ongoing need for innovation in imaging and modeling techniques to make them more efficient and accessible.

Once a comprehensive foot model is established, the subsequent stage involves creating a detailed mesh for the model's volume. This meshing process requires careful consideration of the various regions within the model, as each area may necessitate different types of element geometries that are specifically tailored to its unique characteristics. For instance, in two-dimensional FE models, common element geometries include triangular and quadrilateral shapes. These elements are favored for their simplicity and effectiveness in capturing the geometry of the foot's outline and surface attributes. In contrast, three-dimensional FE models typically utilize tetrahedral or hexahedral elements, which are adept at representing complex volumetric shapes and are crucial for accurately simulating the foot's internal structures [25–27]. A key aspect of meshing is mesh density, which refers to the number of elements within the FE model. The density of the mesh plays a critical role in determining the accuracy and reliability of the simulation results. A higher density mesh, while capable of producing more precise and detailed outcomes, also brings challenges, as it significantly increases computational time and resource consumption [28–31]. This trade-off highlights the importance of optimization in the modeling process. To achieve this balance effectively, it is essential to conduct a mesh convergence study. This study systematically evaluates how variations in mesh density impact the results of the simulations. By incrementally refining the mesh and analyzing the resulting outputs, researchers can identify the optimal mesh configuration that minimizes artifacts and inaccuracies in the simulation data. This process not only allows for higher accuracy but also enhances the reproducibility of the model's findings, ensuring that the simulation results can be reliably used in further research or clinical applications. In conclusion, the development of an accurate and reliable foot model depends on several critical factors. These include the selection of appropriate imaging techniques, the choice of suitable element geometry, and the establishment of optimal mesh density. Each of these components plays a vital role in ensuring that the resulting model not only accurately reflects anatomical precision but also serves as a valuable tool for understanding foot biomechanics and its implications for health and performance. Through this comprehensive approach, researchers can generate insightful analyses that contribute to both scientific knowledge and practical applications in fields such as orthopedics, sports medicine, and rehabilitation [18, 32].

2.3 Material Properties

The development of an accurate foot model for computational analysis is a multifaceted and intricate process that necessitates a thorough understanding of the material properties of the various components that comprise the foot. This modeling process begins with a comprehensive review of existing literature, where researchers have documented the biomechanical properties of different foot structures, such as bones, ligaments, tendons, and soft tissues [33]. By examining previous studies, researchers can identify established norms and variations within foot anatomy and biomechanics. To enhance the accuracy of the model, it is critical to incorporate personalized data obtained from in vivo (conducted in the living body) or in vitro (conducted in controlled laboratory conditions) testing methodologies. These empirical findings provide invaluable insights that ensure the material properties in the model accurately reflect the unique anatomical and biomechanical characteristics of an individual's foot. This level of customization is especially important for patients with conditions like diabetes, which can significantly alter foot mechanics and increase the risk of complications such as ulceration and infections [21]. In an effort to streamline the modeling process and improve computational efficiency, researchers often designate certain elements of the foot model as mechanically stiff. For instance, the ground beneath the foot may be simplified and modeled as a rigid surface, which indicates that it does not deform under the stresses applied during simulations. This strategic simplification reduces the overall complexity of the model while still maintaining the necessary accuracy for realistic assessments and predictions of foot behavior during various activities.

Additionally, the soft tissues of the foot's sole, particularly the plantar fascia, exhibit complex nonlinear viscoelastic properties. These properties can exhibit significant variability depending on the individual's foot condition, with healthy feet demonstrating distinct mechanical behaviors compared to those affected by diabetes or other pathologies [34, 35]. While earlier studies often reported linear mechanical properties for these soft tissues, recent research has recognized the inadequacy of such models. Consequently, there has been a shift toward employing nonlinear material criteria, such as the Ogden hyperelastic model. This model is designed to more accurately represent the intricate and dynamic behavior of plantar soft tissues during a range of loading conditions encountered in everyday activities, ultimately leading to improved predictions of foot function [36, 37]. By focusing on both established literature and incorporating personalized data, this refined approach aims to enhance the precision and applicability of foot models for computational analysis, particularly in clinical contexts where individualized treatment plans are crucial.

Several studies have opted to consolidate the material properties of the foot's various components, including skin, muscles, tendons, and fat pads, into a unified framework known as a lumped foot model. This methodology not only streamlines the analysis but also provides an integrated perspective on the overall mechanical characteristics of the foot. By employing lumped models, researchers have successfully evaluated contact pressures across a variety of conditions, yielding significant insights into how the foot performs during activities such as walking, running, and other athletic movements [38]. In order to develop a robust computational foot model, it is essential to strike a careful balance between a detailed anatomical representation and the simplifications necessary for functional modeling. This balance ensures both computational efficiency and the accuracy of biomechanical analyses. When constructing a realistic geometric model, it becomes imperative to clearly articulate the interactions between different material properties at their contact surfaces. This detail is critical in applications within biomechanics and sports science, where precise modeling can substantially enhance our understanding of human movement dynamics. For instance, when simulating the interaction between the plantar surface of the foot and various ground surfaces, or between the foot and an insole, the realism of the results heavily relies on accurately defining the contact behaviors of these surfaces. This involves the application of friction coefficients, which serve to quantify the resistance encountered during such interactions. Previous research has established that these friction coefficients typically range from 0.3 to 0.6 when analyzing the interaction of the foot's plantar surface with the ground [27, 33]. This range is reflective of the diverse textures and conditions of different surfaces, as well as the myriad types of shoe materials that may be experienced in real-world environments. Ultimately, by integrating detailed anatomical insights with functional modeling techniques, researchers can create more accurate and realistic simulations that not only enhance our comprehension of foot mechanics but also contribute to the development of better footwear, rehabilitation strategies, and athletic performance improvement.

Figure 2.2 presents an illustration of a representative finite element (FE) foot model based on existing literature, and Table 2.1 presents an in-depth summary of

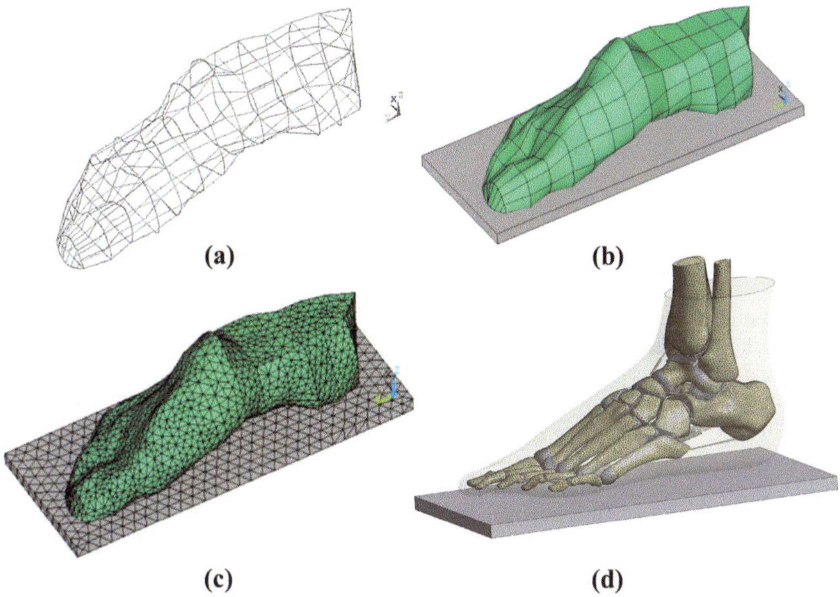

Fig. 2.2 **a** Line wire mesh of foot model, **b** Developed volume model, **c** Meshed foot and ground, and **d** FE model of detailed human foot model. *Reproduced with permission from IOP Science* [1]

pivotal studies in the field of foot modeling, carefully detailing the various structural and material properties evaluated by each study. These investigations shed light on the critical factors that must be carefully considered when creating a foot model that is both accurate and realistic. Each study contributes unique insights, enhancing our understanding of the biomechanical complexities of the foot. To support researchers and practitioners in the modeling process, Fig. 2.3 offers a comprehensive flowchart that outlines a systematic, step-by-step approach to developing and refining a foot model. This structured methodology serves as an essential guide, ensuring that all significant aspects, such as anatomical variations, material behaviors, and dynamic interactions, are thoroughly addressed and integrated into the overall modeling framework. By adhering to this detailed process, researchers can attain a more comprehensive and nuanced understanding of foot dynamics, which is crucial for applications in areas such as orthopedics, sports science, and rehabilitation.

2.4 FEM of Diabetic Foot

FEM has emerged as an invaluable tool in the analysis of human foot biomechanics, particularly in assessing and predicting injury risks associated with various activities such as walking, running, and athletic performance. This advanced computational technique enables researchers to simulate the physical responses of foot structures

Table 2.1 Literature studies on FEM of the human foot and the different material properties. *Reproduced with permission from IOP Science* [1]

Model material	Model components	Elements of the FE model	Remarks
Linear elastic: bones, soft tissue, tendons; viscoelastic: ligaments	28 bones, 3 retinacula, plantar soft tissues (3 layers), 7 ankle ligaments, Achilles tendon	17,503	First notable developed 3D foot model for ankle injury criterion
Linear elastic: bone, cartilage; hyperelastic: soft tissue; truss element: plantar fascia, ligaments	28 bones, soft tissue, plantar fascia, 72 ligaments, cartilages	–	Analyze the response of the plantar fascia in the standing foot condition for different magnitudes of Achilles tendon loading
Linear elastic	Tibia and rigid parts	320,120 hexahedral	Cadaveric foot to develop the FE model of the tibia using CT scans to evaluate the responses under high-force axial loading
Linear elastic: bone, cartilage; truss element: plantar fascia, ligament; hyperelastic: soft tissue	Bones, cartilages, plantar fascia, ligaments, soft tissue	245,782 tetrahedral	3D FE foot model to predict the stress and deformation of internal plantar soft tissue
Linear elastic: bone, skin	Bones, skin, ligaments, plantar fascia	38,870	Analysis of stress distribution by modifying the arch type and estimate the effect of different arch heights
Linear elastic	2D planar model: bones, soft tissue, and phalanges	4,259 quadrilateral	FE foot model to mimic gait cycle using motion-captured data
Linear elastic: bones, cartilage; truss element: ligament; beam element: muscles	28 bones, cartilages, 9 ligaments, 9 muscles	783,000 tetrahedral	FE skeletal foot model to assess the progression of hallux abducto valgus (HAV) forefoot deformity
Linear elastic: bone; truss element: ligament, muscle; hyperelastic: soft tissue	30 bones, ligaments, muscles, soft tissue	–	Estimated fracture risk and the effect of impact velocity on the stress of calcaneus and talus using the FE foot model

(continued)

Table 2.1 (continued)

Model material	Model components	Elements of the FE model	Remarks
Linear elastic	26 bones, plantar fascia, deltoid ligament, Achilles tendon	–	Realistic anatomical foot model
Linear elastic: bone; hyperelastic: soft tissue, elastic force-strain response function: ligament	26 bones, 67 ligaments, soft tissue	450,580 hexahedral	Investigated the injury risk considering different postures of the foot and ankle model
Linear elastic: bone, muscle, cartilage; hyperelastic: tendon, fat tissue	30 cortical bone, 18 trabecular bone, 22 cartilage, plantar fascia, soft tissue, 29 tendons, and muscle	806,475 tetrahedral	Analysis of the tensile forces on the lower limb of the foot and ankle complex
Linear elastic: bone, Implant; axial connector: muscle; truss element: ligament	28 bones, 103 ligaments, plantar fascia, muscles, soft tissue. Tibia/talar and mobile bearing implants	–	Comparison of mechanical performance of the foot model with the implant
Linear elastic: bones; truss element: ligament; hyperelastic: soft tissue	17 bones, ligaments, skin	167,142	FE foot model using MRI scans to analyze the effect of soft tissue stiffness on the plantar pressure distribution
Linear elastic	soft tissue, plantar fascia	23,547 tetrahedral	Custom insole design for stress reduction in diabetic patients
Linear elastic	Soft tissue, plantar fascia	25,784 tetrahedral	Biomechanical modeling of diabetic foot ulceration

to diverse loading conditions and movements, thereby providing crucial insights that can significantly impact preventive medicine and athletic training strategies. A substantial body of research has delved into the complexities of foot biomechanics, with a particular focus on diabetic foot models, which are particularly relevant due to the increasing prevalence of diabetes and its associated complications [39–41]. By utilizing highly detailed and anatomically accurate foot models, researchers can achieve simulations that closely represent the actual biological responses of the foot during various activities. This level of detail is crucial for understanding how different factors, such as pressure distribution, tissue deformation, and stress responses, contribute to the risk of injury and other foot-related disorders [33, 42]. However, despite the significant advantages offered by comprehensive FEM, several challenges complicate its practical application. The intricate nature of these models

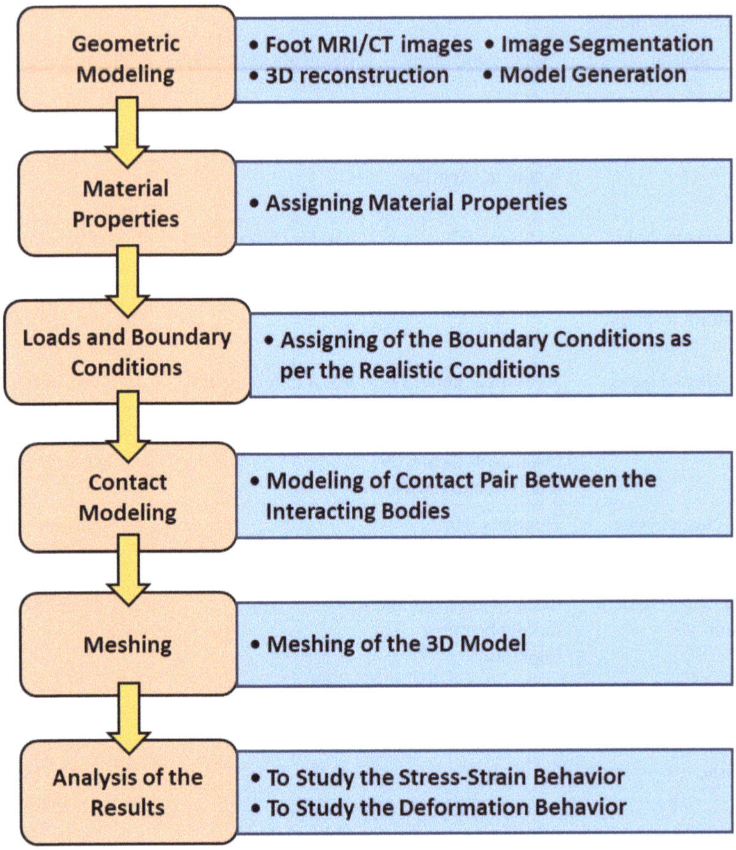

Fig. 2.3 Flowchart for the modeling of the foot model. *Reproduced with permission from IOP Science* [1]

requires substantial time and resources for both development and analysis, which can impede their use in clinical settings. Clinicians and researchers often encounter difficulties in translating these complex models into actionable insights that can be readily applied in time-sensitive healthcare environments. As a result, finding ways to streamline the modeling process and enhance the accessibility of FE analysis in clinical practice remains a critical area for future research and development.

To address the existing gap in our understanding of foot biomechanics, there has been a notable increase in interest in the development of simplified FE models. These models, while lacking some anatomical detail, are designed to deliver reasonable estimates of foot function in shorter analysis times, making them more practical for clinical settings. The primary objective of these streamlined models is to retain vital functional characteristics while significantly reducing computational demands, thus allowing for quicker assessments and applications in patient care [37, 43]. A pertinent illustrative example of this approach can be found in the study conducted by Actis et al. [21], which utilized a two-dimensional model of the foot's sagittal plane. This research specifically targeted the second and third rays of the foot, aiming to investigate the impact of omitting certain anatomical structures, such as the plantar fascia and flexor tendon, on the model's output responses. The study's findings revealed that merging the phalanges of the toes into a single composite bone did not result in significant alterations to the output metrics. This discovery suggests that there are viable pathways for simplification without substantial loss of accuracy, which is encouraging for the future of biomechanical modeling. Although there have not been many studies utilizing FEM of the human foot in the context of specific diseases, such as diabetes, the few existing studies contribute invaluable insights into the underlying biomechanical principles. These insights are critical for advancing our understanding of injury mechanisms, particularly in diabetic populations, and for developing effective prevention strategies tailored to address individual risk factors. By enhancing our comprehension of how foot biomechanics function in varied scenarios, we can better support clinical interventions aimed at preventing injuries and improving overall foot health.

Jacob et al. [44] conducted a comprehensive study focused on developing an intricate three-dimensional (3D) model of the human foot, which incorporated a variety of anatomical components, including bones, ligaments, cartilages, and plantar soft tissues (see Fig. 2.4). This innovative model was constructed using X-ray images obtained from both healthy individuals and diabetic patients, allowing the researchers to systematically contrast the anatomical and functional differences between the two groups. To rigorously analyze the biomechanical behavior of the foot, the researchers simulated the act of walking under quasistatic conditions, paying particular attention to three critical phases: heel strike, midstance, and push-off. The primary objective of this study was to assess the stresses and forces exerted on the diabetic foot in comparison to the normal foot. The researchers focused on nine designated pressure points across both foot models, which were essential in understanding the impact of diabetes on foot biomechanics. The findings from this study revealed that plantar stresses were significantly elevated in the diabetic foot when compared to the normal foot. Specifically, the researchers noted a striking increase in vertical stresses within the plantar region during the critical phases of walking; stress levels surged in the heel region during heel strike and in the forefoot region during the push-off phase. These heightened stress levels indicate a greater risk of injury and complications for individuals with diabetes. In a related investigation, Gefen [18] developed an advanced diabetic foot model aimed at analyzing the loading characteristics of the plantar soft tissues in balanced standing conditions. This study varied the stiffness of the soft tissues to emulate different progression levels of diabetes, recognizing that tissue stiffness can significantly influence foot health. The results demonstrated that contact forces at the first and second metatarsal heads increased dramatically, by 50%. Additionally, internal tissue stresses escalated significantly with an alarming increase of 307%, attributed to the heightened stiffness of the tissues. This finding underscores the severe implications for foot health in diabetic patients, highlighting the risk of developing ulcers and other complications due to increased stress on the plantar tissues.

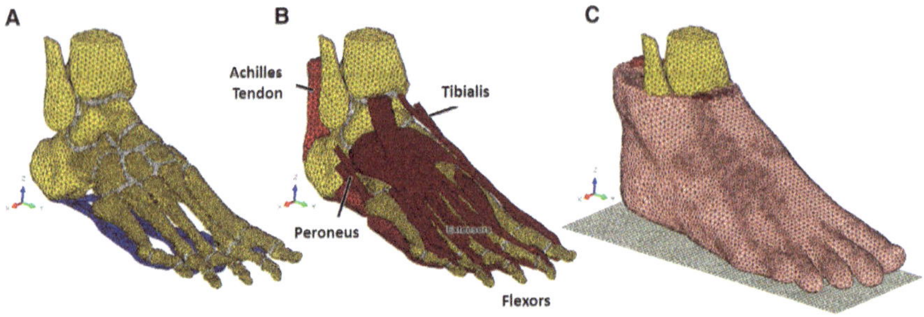

Fig. 2.4 Tissue layers of the finite element model. **a** Skeleton + fascia, **b** Skeleton + muscle/ tendons, and **c** Skeleton + soft tissue + ground. *Reproduced with permission from IOP Science* [1]

Further contributing to this area of research, Thomas et al. [36] developed a 3D foot model that integrated variations in the thickness and stiffness of soft tissues to simulate and compare the conditions experienced by healthy and diabetic feet during the push-off phase of walking. Their simulation revealed an increase in both normal and shear stresses in the plantar region when exposed to diabetic conditions, with stress levels rising by 52.3% and 53.6%, respectively. These increased stress levels can further exacerbate the risk of injury for diabetic individuals, indicating a need for targeted interventions and preventive strategies. Gu et al. [45] investigated the impact of heel skin stiffness on the biomechanics of the hindfoot, particularly during the heel strike phase of walking. Their research findings indicated that increased skin stiffness among diabetic patients led to a 14.2% rise in peak plantar pressure in the heel region, highlighting the compounded risks that diabetic patients face during ambulation. This increased pressure can lead to skin breakdown and ulceration, emphasizing the need for careful management of foot health in this population. Lastly, Chen et al. [24] modeled a three-dimensional foot to scrutinize its performance under balanced standing conditions, specifically aiming to differentiate between normal and diabetic scenarios. Their results revealed a concerning threefold increase in internal stresses compared to normal conditions, which correlates with an elevated risk of ulceration in the plantar region. This significant finding highlights the urgent need for healthcare providers to monitor and address the biomechanical challenges faced by individuals with diabetes in order to prevent serious complications and improve overall foot health.

Various researchers have increasingly recognized the importance of exploring alternative methods for diabetic foot modeling that extend beyond traditional techniques. There is a growing consensus on the need for the development of geometrically simplified models, which, despite their reduced complexity, can still provide outcomes comparable to more intricate models. These simplified models offer the advantage of enabling faster and more efficient simulations of diabetic conditions, making them particularly valuable in a clinical setting where timeliness can be critical. While there is still some uncertainty regarding the precision of these simplified models in generating accurate, patient-specific estimates for various parameters, such as pressure distribution, tissue stress, and ulcer formation, their advantages in terms of construction and computational efficiency are significant. These models facilitate a deeper understanding of biomechanical properties and enhance finite element simulation techniques, serving as crucial tools for researchers investigating the effects of different therapeutic interventions on DFUs [46, 47]. By utilizing these simplified models, researchers can gain important insights into the underlying mechanisms that contribute to the pathophysiology of diabetic foot complications. Moreover, such models pave the way for the development of improved therapeutic strategies tailored to individual patients. Ultimately, the continued refinement and application of these models have the potential to lead to better management of DFUs, thereby improving patient outcomes and quality of life.

2.5 FEM of DFUs

Investigating the physical factors associated with foot ulcers in humans poses significant challenges, particularly when attempting to obtain direct measurements in in vivo (within a living organism) or in vitro (in a controlled environment outside of a living organism) settings. FEM serves as a powerful computational method for estimating the stresses and strains that occur in tissues affected by ulcers, thereby offering valuable insights into their development and progression. Numerous experimental studies have demonstrated considerable differences in both the thickness and stiffness of plantar soft tissues when comparing diabetic individuals to their healthy counterparts. For instance, Guiotto et al. [48] conducted a detailed examination of the morphological changes that take place in the foot as ulcers develop. Their research revealed that these changes are closely linked to the mechanical stresses exerted on the deeper tissues within the plantar pad, which serves as a critical shock absorber during weight-bearing activities. Individuals suffering from diabetic neuropathy, a condition commonly associated with diabetes that affects nerve function, experience heightened mechanical stress in specific areas of the foot, such as the calcaneus (the heel bone) and the metatarsal heads (the long bones located at the ball of the foot). The excessive stress in these regions plays a significant role in the onset and exacerbation of foot ulcers, as detailed by prior studies [11].

In a subsequent study, Guiotto et al. [49] advanced the understanding of foot biomechanics by developing a subject-specific foot model using high-fidelity MRI data. This comprehensive model encompassed the anatomical structures, including bones, skin, and cartilage, of both a diabetic patient with neuropathic foot complications and a healthy individual for comparative analysis. The researchers conducted dynamic simulations based on gait data collected from a cohort of ten participants, which included both neuropathic and healthy patients. They measured peak pressure values and overall pressure distribution across various regions of the foot during different phases of walking. Upon analyzing the results, the researchers noted a discrepancy of approximately 20% between the numerical outcomes generated by the FEM and the experimental results obtained from the foot models of individuals with neuropathy. This difference underscores the inherent complexity of accurately modeling biological systems while illustrating the potential of FEM as an invaluable tool in enhancing our understanding of the biomechanical environment of the diabetic foot. The application of FEM in producing detailed three-dimensional simulations of the human foot, particularly in relation to diabetic neuropathy, offers significant insights into the underlying mechanisms that contribute to foot ulcer formation. This understanding is crucial for the development of effective and targeted prevention and treatment strategies. By improving our comprehension of these mechanisms, healthcare providers can ultimately enhance patient care and improve the overall quality of life for individuals affected by DFUs. To develop a detailed 3D model of the human foot, the process begins by capturing the geometry of both the foot's skeletal structure and its surrounding soft tissues through the reconstruction of MRI images (refer to Fig. 2.5). This process involves advanced imaging techniques that provide high-resolution insights into the intricate anatomy of the foot. By understanding how these soft tissue characteristics interact with the skeletal framework, we can better assess and manage foot health, particularly in individuals with diabetes [34, 50].

Finite element research focused on diabetic foot conditions has quantified the relationship between peak pressure in the plantar region and changes in the composition of the plantar soft tissues, specifically their thickness and stiffness. These findings, drawn from both two-dimensional and three-dimensional modeling approaches, underscore the necessity of incorporating tissue deformation into foot health assessments. This is especially important for diabetic patients, who are prone to complications related to foot ulcers [18, 36]. In identifying critical areas for stress distribution, researchers have determined specific locations where internal stresses reach

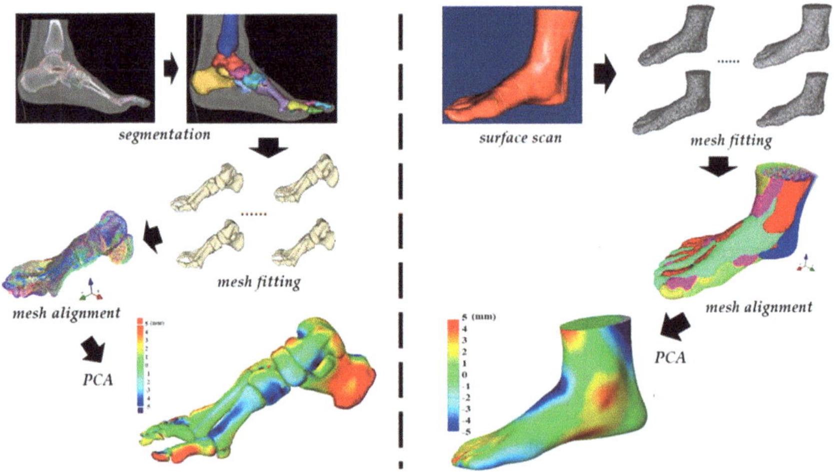

Fig. 2.5 An outline of the workflow in the statistical shape modeling of foot bones (left) and surface (right) shapes. Steps of segmentation (bone) or surface scan (surface), mesh fitting, mesh alignment, and principal component analysis (PCA). *Reproduced with permission from IOP Science* [1]

their maximum. Notably, these high-stress regions are located near the metatarsophalangeal joints, at the heads of the metatarsals, and beneath the third and fourth metatarsal heads. Such stress concentrations typically occur at the midpoint between the underlying bony structures and the plantar surface of the foot. Understanding these dynamics is crucial because they can significantly increase the risk of injury or ulceration, particularly in diabetic patients who may experience reduced sensation and circulation in the foot [18]. In a significant advancement within this field, Chanda and Unnikrishnan [51] developed a comprehensive foot model aimed at a detailed analysis of stress distribution in the plantar region, with a specific focus on ulcers of varying shapes, both regular and irregular, typically found at the heel. Their innovative methodology involved utilizing the precise foot coordinates of a human subject to construct a full-scale, anatomically accurate model of the foot. This approach enabled a more realistic simulation of real-world conditions, enhancing the reliability of their findings. Through meticulous analysis of the stress distribution patterns in their model, Chanda and Unnikrishnan [51] proposed several targeted interventions to mitigate the risk of ulcer development and progression. Among these recommendations was the use of specialized insoles designed to better distribute pressure across the foot, thereby alleviating stress in the most vulnerable areas. These insights and recommendations are vital for improving the management of diabetic foot conditions and ultimately enhancing patient care, helping to prevent severe complications that could lead to amputations or decreased quality of life for affected individuals [52, 53].

References

1. Singh G, Chanda A (2024) Finite element modeling of diabetic foot: a state-of-the-art review. Eng Res Express 6:012507
2. Chhikara K, Singh G, Gupta S, Chanda A (2022) Progress of additive manufacturing in fabrication of foot orthoses for diabetic patients: A review. Ann 3D Print Med 8, 100085
3. Gupta S et al (2023) Diabot: development of a diabetic foot pressure tracking device. J 6, 32–47
4. Bose D, Singh G, Gupta S, Chanda A (2024) Development of a novel customized insole for effective pressure offloading in diabetic patients. Prosthesis 6:341–356
5. Singh G, Chanda A (2021) Mechanical properties of whole-body soft human tissues: a review. Biomed Mater 16:062004
6. Ratchev S, Liu S, Huang W, Becker AA (2006) An advanced FEA based force induced error compensation strategy in milling. Int J Mach Tools Manuf 46:542–551
7. Engelke K, van Rietbergen B, Zysset P (2016) FEA to measure bone strength: a review. Clin Rev Bone Miner Metab. 14:26–37
8. Belhocine A, Abdullah OI (2020) Design and thermomechanical finite element analysis of frictional contact mechanism on automotive disc brake assembly. J Fail Anal Prev 20:270–301
9. Belhocine A, Abdullah OI (2022) Finite element analysis (FEA) of frictional contact phenomenon on vehicle braking system. Mech Based Des Struct. 1–36. https://doi.org/10.1080/15397734.2020.1787843.
10. Singh G, Chanda A (2022) Biomechanical modeling of progressive wound healing: A computational study. Biomed Eng Adv. 4:100055
11. Erdemir A, Guess TM, Halloran J, Tadepalli SC, Morrison TM (2012) Considerations for reporting finite element analysis studies in biomechanics. J Biomech 45:625–633

12. Abdel-Nasser YA (2013) Frontal crash simulation of vehicles against lighting columns using FEM. Alexandria Eng J. 52:295–299
13. Murni NS, Dambatta MS, Yeap SK, Froemming GRA, Hermawan H (2015) Cytotoxicity evaluation of biodegradable Zn–3Mg alloy toward normal human osteoblast cells. Mater Sci Eng C 49:560–566
14. Filardi V (2018) Finite element analysis of the foot: Stress and displacement shielding. J Orthop 15:974–979
15. Jain ML, Govind Dhande S, Vyas NS (2011) Virtual modeling of an ankle foot orthosis for correction of foot abnormality. Robot Comput Integr Manuf. 27, 257–260
16. Sijbrandij ES, Van Gils APG, De Lange EE (2002) Overuse and sports-related injuries of the ankle and hind foot: MR imaging findings. Eur J Radiol 43:45–56
17. Dixon SJ, Creaby MW, Allsopp AJ (2006) Comparison of static and dynamic biomechanical measures in military recruits with and without a history of third metatarsal stress fracture. Clin Biomech 21:412–419
18. Gefen A (2003) Plantar soft tissue loading under the medial metatarsals in the standing diabetic foot. Med Eng Phys 25:491–499
19. Erdemir A, Viveiros ML, Ulbrecht JS, Cavanagh PR (2006) An inverse finite-element model of heel-pad indentation. J Biomech 39:1279–1286
20. Thomas VJ, Patil KM, Radhakrishnan S (2004) Three-dimensional stress analysis for the mechanics of plantar ulcers in diabetic neuropathy. Med Biol Eng Comput 42:230–235
21. Actis RL et al (2006) Numerical simulation of the plantar pressure distribution in the diabetic foot during the push-off stance. Med Biol Eng Comput 44:653–663
22. Goske S, Erdemir A, Petre M, Budhabhatti S, Cavanagh PR (2006) Reduction of plantar heel pressures: Insole design using finite element analysis. J Biomech 39:2363–2370
23. Cheung JTM, Zhang M (2005) A 3-dimensional finite element model of the human foot and ankle for insole design. Arch Phys Med Rehabil 86:353–358
24. Chen WM, Lee T, Lee PVS, Lee JW, Lee SJ (2010) Effects of internal stress concentrations in plantar soft-tissue—A preliminary three-dimensional finite element analysis. Med Eng Phys 32:324–331
25. Budhabhatti SP et al (2007) Finite element modeling of the first ray of the foot: a tool for the design of interventions. J Biomech Eng 129:750–756
26. Chen WM, Park J, Park SB, Shim VPW, Lee T (2012) Role of gastrocnemius–soleus muscle in forefoot force transmission at heel rise—A 3D finite element analysis. J Biomech 45:1783–1789
27. Tadepalli SC, Erdemir A, Cavanagh PR (2011) Comparison of hexahedral and tetrahedral elements in finite element analysis of the foot and footwear. J Biomech 44:2337–2343
28. Gupta V, Chanda A (2022) Biomechanics of skin grafts: effect of pattern size, spacing and orientation. Eng Res Express 4:015006
29. Chanda A, Unnikrishnan V, Richter HE, Lockhart ME (2016) A biofidelic computational model of the female pelvic system to understand effect of bladder fill and progressive vaginal tissue stiffening due to prolapse on anterior vaginal wall. Int J Numer Method Biomed Eng. 32:e02767
30. Gupta S, Chanda A (2023) Biomechanical modeling of footwear-fluid-floor interaction during slips. J Biomech 156:111690
31. Gupta V, Gupta S, Chanda A (2022) Expansion potential of skin grafts with novel rotating-triangle-shaped auxetic incisions. Emerg Mater Res. 11:406–414
32. Lemmon D, Shiang TY, Hashmi A, Ulbrecht JS, Cavanagh PR (1997) The effect of insoles in therapeutic footwear—A finite element approach. J Biomech 30:615–620
33. Isvilanonda V, Dengler E, Iaquinto JM, Sangeorzan BJ, Ledoux WR (2012) Finite element analysis of the foot: Model validation and comparison between two common treatments of the clawed hallux deformity. Clin Biomech 27:837–844
34. Pai S, Ledoux WR (2010) The compressive mechanical properties of diabetic and non-diabetic plantar soft tissue. J Biomech 43:1754–1760
35. Petre M, Erdemir A, Panoskaltsis VP, Spirka TA, Cavanagh PR (2013) Optimization of nonlinear hyperelastic coefficients for foot tissues using a magnetic resonance imaging deformation experiment. J Biomech Eng. 135

36. Thomas VJ, Patil KM, Radhakrishnan S (2004) Three-dimensional stress analysis for the mechanics of plantar ulcers in diabetic neuropathy. Med Biol Eng Comput 422 42, 230–235.
37. Yarnitzky G, Yizhar Z, Gefen A (2006) Real-time subject-specific monitoring of internal deformations and stresses in the soft tissues of the foot: A new approach in gait analysis. J Biomech 39:2673–2689
38. Cheung JTM, Zhang M, Leung AKL, Fan YB (2005) Three-dimensional finite element analysis of the foot during standing—a material sensitivity study. J Biomech 38:1045–1054
39. Smolen C, Quenneville CE (2017) A finite element model of the foot/ankle to evaluate injury risk in various postures. Ann Biomed Eng 45:1993–2008
40. Wang Y, Li Z, Wong DWC, Cheng CK, Zhang M (2018) Finite element analysis of biomechanical effects of total ankle arthroplasty on the foot. J Orthop Transl. 12:55–65
41. Wang H, Brown SR (2017) The effects of total ankle replacement on ankle joint mechanics during walking. J Sport Heal Sci. 6:340–345
42. Fernandez JW, Ul Haque MZ, Hunter PJ, Mithraratne K (2012) Mechanics of the foot Part 1: A continuum framework for evaluating soft tissue stiffening in the pathologic foot. Int J Numer Method Biomed Eng. 28, 1056–1070
43. Actis RL et al (2008) Multi-plug insole design to reduce peak plantar pressure on the diabetic foot during walking. Med Biol Eng Comput 46:363–371
44. Jacob S, Patil MK (1999) Stress analysis in three-dimensional foot models of normal and diabetic neuropathy. Front Med Biol Eng 9:211–227
45. Gu Y, Li J, Ren X, Lake MJ, Zeng Y (2010) Heel skin stiffness effect on the hind foot biomechanics during heel strike. Ski. Res. Technol. 16:291–296
46. Singh G, Gupta S, Chanda A (2021) Biomechanical modelling of diabetic foot ulcers: A computational study. J Biomech 127:110699
47. Gupta S, Singh G, Chanda A (2021) Prediction of diabetic foot ulcer progression: a computational study. Biomed Phys Eng Express 7:065020
48. Guiotto A et al (2013) The role of foot morphology on foot function in diabetic subjects with or without neuropathy. Gait Posture 37:603–610
49. Guiotto A, Sawacha Z, Guarneri G, Avogaro A, Cobelli C (2014) 3D finite element model of the diabetic neuropathic foot: A gait analysis driven approach. J Biomech 47:3064–3071
50. Klaesner JW, Hastings MK, Zou D, Lewis C, Mueller MJ (2002) Plantar tissue stiffness in patients with diabetes mellitus and peripheral neuropathy. Arch Phys Med Rehabil 83:1796–1801
51. Chanda A, Unnikrishnan V (2018) Novel insole design for diabetic foot ulcer management. Proc Inst Mech Eng Part H J Eng Med 232, 1182–1195
52. Singh G, Lamba A, Chanda A (2024) Role of additive manufacturing for the management of diabetic foot ulcers. In Addit Manuf Biomed Appl 19–38 (Springer, Singapore). https://doi.org/10.1007/978-981-97-5456-4_2
53. Singh G, Bose D, Chanda A (2025) Development and testing of a novel diabetic orthosis for plantar pressure reduction. Facta Univ Ser Mech Eng. https://doi.org/10.22190/FUME240725044S

Chapter 3
Computational Modeling of Diabetic Ulcers Across Different Foot Types

3.1 Introduction

Diabetic foot ulcers (DFUs) represent a multifaceted medical condition often initiated by irregular pressure distribution on the foot, which can lead to the breakdown of the plantar fascia, a critical structure that supports the arch of the foot. This breakdown of the fascia increases the risk of ulceration, a serious complication for those living with diabetes [1–3]. Despite substantial research exploring diabetic ulcers from various medical and treatment perspectives, there remains a significant gap in the comprehensive understanding of the biomechanical factors that contribute to their development. The primary variables influencing ulceration are the location, size, and depth of the ulcer. Ulcers can be predominantly classified into two main categories based on location: plantar regions, which encompass the bottom of the foot, and non-plantar regions [4, 5]. Within the plantar areas, ulcers frequently occur in the forefoot and hindfoot regions, which are more susceptible to pressure and trauma. Comparatively, the midfoot experiences a lower incidence of ulceration. While the majority of DFUs are classified as superficial, about 15% can penetrate the underlying tendons, which poses an increased risk of infection and complications. Furthermore, approximately 17% of ulcers may extend deep enough to impact the underlying bone, making the condition more severe and requiring more intensive intervention [6–9]. When evaluating the size of an ulcer, both its surface area and depth must be assessed. However, accurately determining the depth can be particularly challenging due to the irregular characteristics and varying shapes of the ulcer. In addition to anatomical challenges, extrinsic factors such as poorly fitting footwear, often too tight or excessively worn, and preexisting foot deformities, like bunions or hammertoes, can lead to increased plantar pressure. This exacerbates the risk of developing DFUs and can intensify their severity, highlighting the need for proper footwear and foot care management in diabetic patients. In summary, understanding the complex interplay of biomechanical factors, ulcer characteristics, and external influences is crucial for developing effective prevention and treatment strategies for DFUs [10–12].

A. Chanda and G. Singh, *Diabetic Foot Ulcer*, Biomedical Materials for Multi-functional Applications, https://doi.org/10.1007/978-981-95-2484-6_3

Flatfoot, also known as pes planus, is a condition where the arch of the foot collapses, causing the entire flexed plantar surface to make contact with the ground. This common foot deformity can lead to various complications, especially concerning overall foot health and mobility. When flatfoot is present, the abnormal load distribution across the foot can result in excessive wear on certain areas, leading to pain and discomfort during standing and movement. The causes of flatfoot are diverse and can include genetic predisposition, which means that some individuals may inherit a tendency toward this condition. Repetitive strain on the plantar tissues from activities such as running or standing for extended periods can also contribute to its development [13, 14]. Additionally, weak arches can be a significant factor, making the foot less capable of absorbing shock. Injuries to the foot or ankle may further exacerbate the risk of developing flatfoot. It is noteworthy that flatfoot is particularly prevalent among individuals who are overweight or obese, which can complicate the management of related health conditions, especially diabetes. The additional weight can increase the stress placed on the foot, worsening the effects of abnormal loading patterns [15]. Moreover, the irregular distribution of forces associated with flatfoot can lead to excessive supination, where the foot rolls outward, and excessive pronation, where the foot rolls inward. Both of these biomechanical changes can create added stress on the foot's structure, potentially resulting in foot pain, joint issues, and conditions such as plantar fasciitis. These biomechanical alterations are critical, as they can significantly influence the progression of DFUs [16]. Understanding the mechanics of flatfoot and its impact on weight distribution is essential for developing effective prevention and treatment strategies. A comprehensive approach to foot care, including proper footwear, orthotic supports, and regular monitoring, can help mitigate the risks associated with flatfoot, particularly for individuals managing diabetes.

Biomechanical studies on diabetic ulcers encounter significant experimental challenges, primarily due to ethical considerations and stringent biosafety regulations [17]. These challenges often hinder direct experimentation involving human subjects or animal models. To mitigate such issues, researchers have employed the finite element modeling (FEM), a sophisticated computational technique widely utilized to create detailed models of the human foot. FEM allows for the analysis of complex mechanical interactions and stress distributions, thus facilitating a deeper understanding of the mechanics governing diabetic ulcers. A particularly insightful study conducted by Chanda and Unnikrishnan [18] investigated the impact of two specific ulcer locations, the forefoot and the heel, on plantar pressure distribution using a computational model of a healthy human foot. Their research revealed that when evaluating circular ulcer geometries, the peak stress experienced on the walls of an ulcer at these locations was amplified by a factor of two compared to a diabetic foot lacking any ulcers. This significant increase in stress emphasizes the critical influence of both the location and geometric characteristics of ulcers on diabetic foot health outcomes. By simultaneously considering both ulcer locations within their simulations, the study provided valuable insights into how plantar stress is distributed across the entire foot, helping to elucidate the mechanical factors contributing to ulcer development. However, it is essential to recognize that this study also had limitations. It focused solely on two ulcer sites and did not consider the variability associated with different foot arch types, nor did it investigate the independent effects of varying ulcer sizes and depths on stress distribution. Such factors could significantly influence therapeutic strategies and the overall management of diabetic foot complications, highlighting the need for further research to capture a more comprehensive view of these dynamics.

In this study, we developed a comprehensive full-scale model of a human foot to examine the effects of various factors associated with diabetic ulcers, specifically focusing on the location, size, and depth of these ulcers in the plantar region. Diabetic ulcers are a significant concern for individuals with diabetes, and understanding their impact on foot health is crucial for effective prevention and treatment. To broaden the analysis, we also utilized a computationally modified flat foot model. This allowed us to simulate and assess how identical ulcer conditions could influence the foot's structural integrity and functional dynamics in individuals with flat foot. Flat foot conditions can alter weight distribution and pressure points, which may affect ulcer development and healing. By conducting a comparative analysis of the results obtained from both the full-scale foot model and the flat foot model, we aimed to uncover the similarities and differences in the resulting biomechanical effects on the plantar surface. This dual approach not only enhances our understanding of the mechanics behind diabetic ulcers but also sheds light on the intricate relationships between foot structure, ulcer characteristics, and potential treatment strategies. Overall, our findings provide critical insights that could inform clinical practices aimed at preventing and managing diabetic ulcers effectively.

3.2 Materials and Methods

3.2.1 Geometrical Modeling

Measurements of the X, Y, and Z Cartesian coordinates were obtained using three calibrated rulers to develop an accurate model of the right foot of a human subject, as illustrated in Fig. 3.1. To capture the foot's complex shape and dimensions in detail, a total of 301 marked points were accurately recorded around its contours. To maintain both consistency and precision during the data collection process, the subject's foot was carefully secured inside a specially designed box while they remained seated in a stable position. This setup significantly minimized any potential movement that could compromise the accuracy of the measurements. Moreover, five critical reference points were systematically designated on the subject's foot: two points on the toes, two on the midfoot, and one on the hindfoot. These reference points were not only labeled but also rigorously cross-checked for accuracy every 15 min to ensure the reliability and integrity of the data collected over time. Once the measurements were gathered, the recorded points were rounded to one decimal place for uniformity,

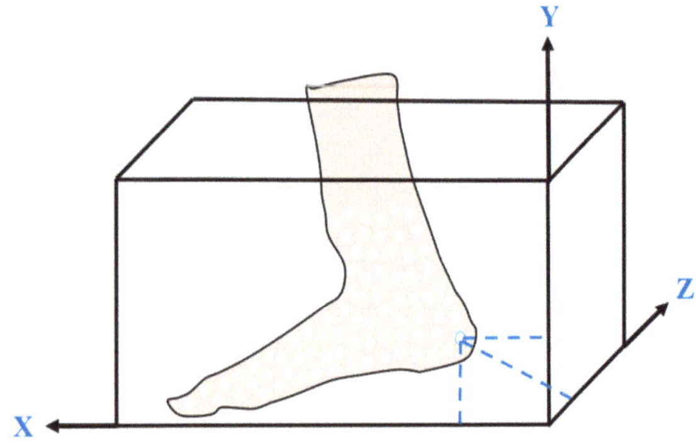

Fig. 3.1 Schematic of Cartesian coordinates measurement to record 301 points on the foot. *Reproduced with permission from Elsevier* [19]

facilitating easier analysis and comparison. These points were then manually plotted in Ansys APDL 2019R2, a powerful engineering simulation software. This software allowed for the creation of a wire mesh representation by interconnecting the points with lines and splines, resulting in a comprehensive and detailed visualization of the foot's intricate structure. This detailed approach not only illustrates the contour of the foot but also serves as a foundation for further biomechanical analysis and modeling.

To develop a comprehensive model of a flat foot, several modifications were implemented on the original normal foot model. The process began by adjusting the arch coordinates, which involved the systematic removal of specific geometric elements integral to the foot's structure. This included deleting the volumes associated with the arch itself, as well as removing the corresponding areas and the lines that connected these areas. Adjustments were made to key points in the model to accurately replicate the unique characteristics of a flat foot, as illustrated in Fig. 3.2. To create detailed areas from the lines, a manual bottom-up approach was utilized. This method allowed for precise control over the geometric configurations, ensuring that the resultant areas were correctly defined. Once these areas were established, they were subsequently combined to form three-dimensional volumes representing both the normal and flat foot models, as depicted in Fig. 3.3. In addition to modifying the foot structures, a direct modeling approach was employed to construct a customized ground surface beneath each foot model. This ground layer was designed to maintain a uniform thickness of 10 mm, which is critical for simulating realistic interactions between the foot and various surfaces. The carefully crafted ground surface is essential for conducting thorough analyses of foot biomechanics, as it provides insights into how different foot shapes respond to different types of terrain and load-bearing conditions. This level of detail ensures that the models are not only accurate in their representations but also effective for further biomechanical studies and applications.

In this study, we conducted a thorough review of existing literature to identify five distinct ulcer sites that are frequently observed in clinical practice. These sites include two on the forefoot: the hallux (commonly known as the big toe) and the first metatarsal bone. Additionally, we selected one site located on the midfoot, specifically targeting the lateral midfoot area. Lastly, there are two ulcer sites identified

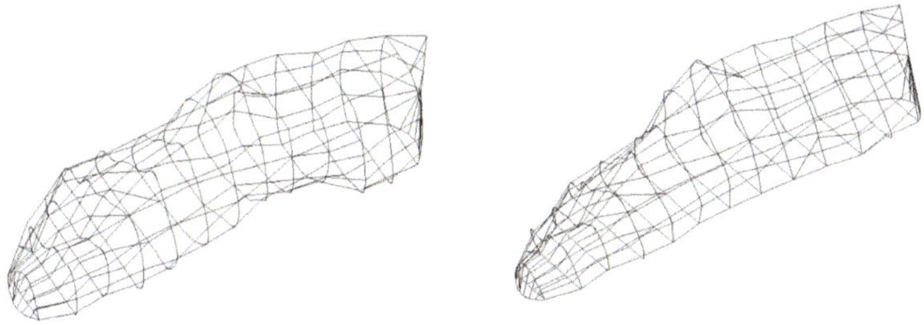

(A) (B)

Fig. 3.2 Wire mesh model in Ansys showing: **a** normal foot and **b** flatfoot

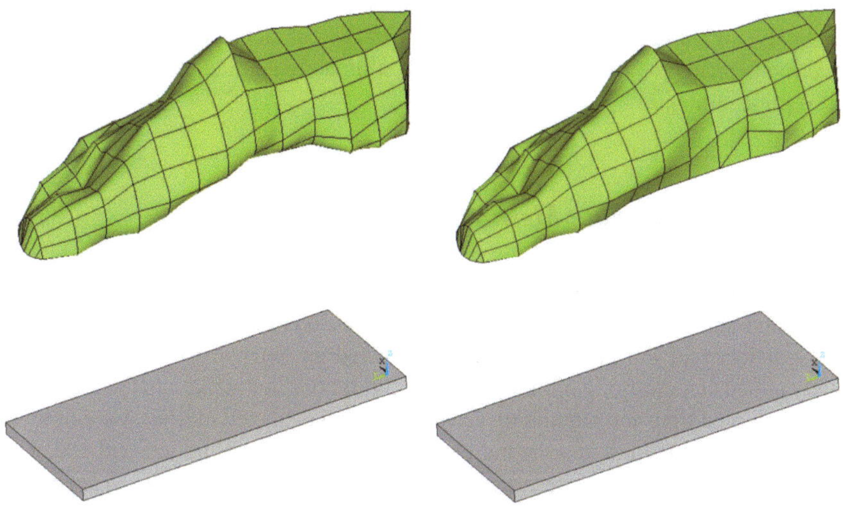

(A) (B)

Fig. 3.3 **a** Normal foot model with the custom ground and **b** Flat foot model with the custom ground. *Reproduced with permission from Elsevier* [19]

on the hindfoot: the medial heel and the lateral heel [18, 20, 21]. The rationale for choosing these specific sites was grounded in their prevalence and clinical significance in patients with diabetic ulcers, which are a common and serious complication of diabetes. To simulate the clinical conditions of these ulcers more accurately, we modeled two different depths of ulceration: a superficial depth of 5 mm, which represents more moderate ulcers that affect the upper layers of the skin, and a deeper depth of 8 mm, which extends down to the fascia and signifies more severe ulcers that can lead to increased complications [22, 23]. In addition to exploring different depths, we also systematically modeled circular ulcers at each of the selected sites, using diameters of 10 mm and 16 mm. This variability in size allows us to better understand the impact of ulcer size on healing and management strategies. By examining these characteristics, we aim to provide insights that can improve clinical outcomes for individuals suffering from diabetic ulcers.

Figure 3.4 presents a detailed visual representation of five common ulcer locations identified on a normal foot model. To enhance our understanding, these same ulceration sites were also indicated on a flat foot model, facilitating a comprehensive investigation into how different foot structures influence ulcer behavior and healing processes. A total of twenty-foot models were developed for this study. Each model incorporates the five ulcer sites, and we varied the experimental parameters by including two sizes of ulcers (10 mm and 16 mm) and two depths (5 mm and 8 mm). This extensive and varied modeling approach not only allows for a thorough examination of the incidence of diabetic ulcers but also provides valuable insights into how foot morphology, differences between normal and flat foot, affect the healing process. By analyzing these models, we aim to uncover critical factors that contribute to the development and recovery of diabetic ulcers, ultimately guiding better treatment and prevention strategies.

3.2.2 *Finite Element Meshing*

The volumes of the foot models were divided into tetrahedral elements to facilitate a detailed and comprehensive analysis of their behaviors. To ensure the accuracy and efficiency of our simulations, we conducted an extensive mesh convergence study aimed at identifying optimal mesh configurations that strike a balance between computational time and simulation accuracy. For all analyzed meshes, we employed a higher-order quadratic tetrahedral element known as the 20-node Solid 186. This choice was intentional, as these elements possess superior capabilities in accurately representing complex geometric features and are particularly effective at capturing the significant deflections and strains that occur during interactions between the foot and the ground [24]. In our mesh convergence analysis, we focused on a standard normal foot model and created four distinct types of meshes, each differing in element count (Fig. 3.5). The meshes included a coarse mesh with 2,645 elements, a semi-coarse mesh with 7,551 elements, a fine mesh with 11,144 elements, and a very fine mesh featuring 25,784 elements. This diverse range of mesh densities allowed us to systematically assess the relationship between mesh granularity and the resulting simulation accuracy, as well as the computational resources required for each configuration. Furthermore, to accurately model the interaction between the foot model and the ground surface, we implemented a contact pair mechanism. This mechanism will be described in detail in the following section, highlighting its importance in ensuring realistic simulations of foot–ground interactions.

For the flat foot model, five different types of tetrahedral-free mapped meshes were developed to conduct a mesh convergence study (see Fig. 3.6). These meshes vary in coarseness and include: very coarse (1,789 elements), coarse (6,715 elements), semi-fine (11,227 elements), fine (15,962 elements), and very fine (21,459 elements).

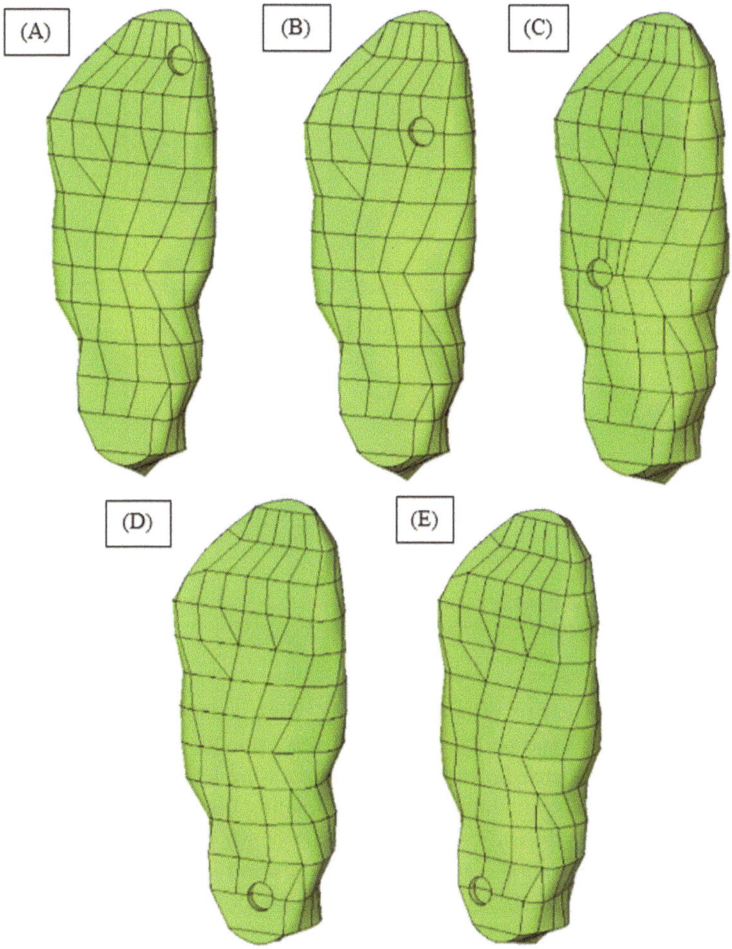

Fig. 3.4 Ulcer site representation on the plantar region of the normal foot at: **a** Hallux, **b** First metatarsal, **c** Lateral midfoot, **d** Medial heel, and **e** Lateral heel. *Reproduced with permission from Elsevier* [19]

3.2.3 Loads and Boundary Conditions

There is a significant variation in foot loads and boundary conditions among individuals, influenced by several factors including foot measurements, body weight, and height. These differences are critical as they affect how pressure is distributed across the foot during various activities, such as walking or running. Research in this area has quantified foot pressure, revealing that the normal forces exerted by individuals with different body weights generally fall within a range of 0.1 to 0.3 MPa [18]. This range reflects the stress experienced by the foot's surface and highlights the importance of considering individual differences when analyzing foot mechanics

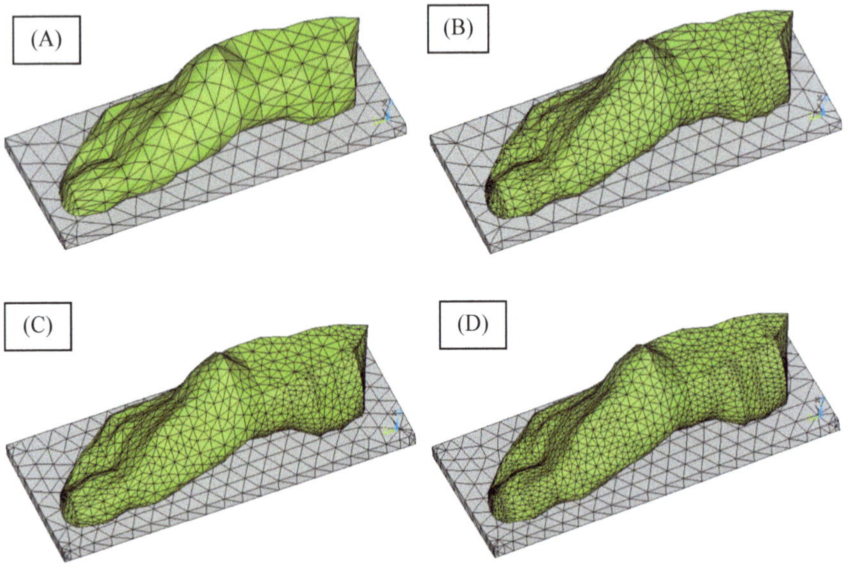

Fig. 3.5 Normal foot model and ground meshes: **a** Coarse, **b** Semi-coarse, **c** Fine, and **d** Very fine. *Reproduced with permission from Elsevier* [19]

and designing footwear or orthotic solutions. Understanding these variations can help improve comfort and performance for diverse populations.

In this study, we focused on analyzing foot pressure loads, selecting a consistent upper limit of 0.3 MPa to simulate extreme loading conditions that may occur in various high-impact scenarios, such as sports or heavy physical activities, as illustrated in Fig. 3.7. This choice was made to understand how the foot behaves under significant stress, which can be critical for designing footwear and orthotic devices. To ensure a robust analysis, particularly for the mesh convergence study, we incorporated three different pressure loads: 0.1 MPa, 0.2 MPa, and 0.3 MPa. By using this range of loads, we aimed to capture a comprehensive view of the maximum von Mises stresses that could develop at the plantar surface of the foot. This method allowed us to accurately identify the optimal mesh configuration required for subsequent detailed analyses, ensuring that our findings would be reliable and applicable in practical settings. The simulations were conducted under carefully controlled conditions, with the bottom surface of the ground fixed in all degrees of freedom. This approach helped maintain stability during the simulation process, providing a solid foundation to accurately assess the foot's response to pressure loads. A contact pair was established between the top surface of the ground and the bottom surface of the foot model. By representing this interaction accurately, we aimed to closely mimic real-life loading scenarios. To further enhance the realism of our simulations, we selected a flexible contact pair defined by a penetration tolerance of 0.1 and a normal penalty stiffness of 1. This choice was crucial for mimicking realistic movements and deformations that occur during foot loading, allowing for a more

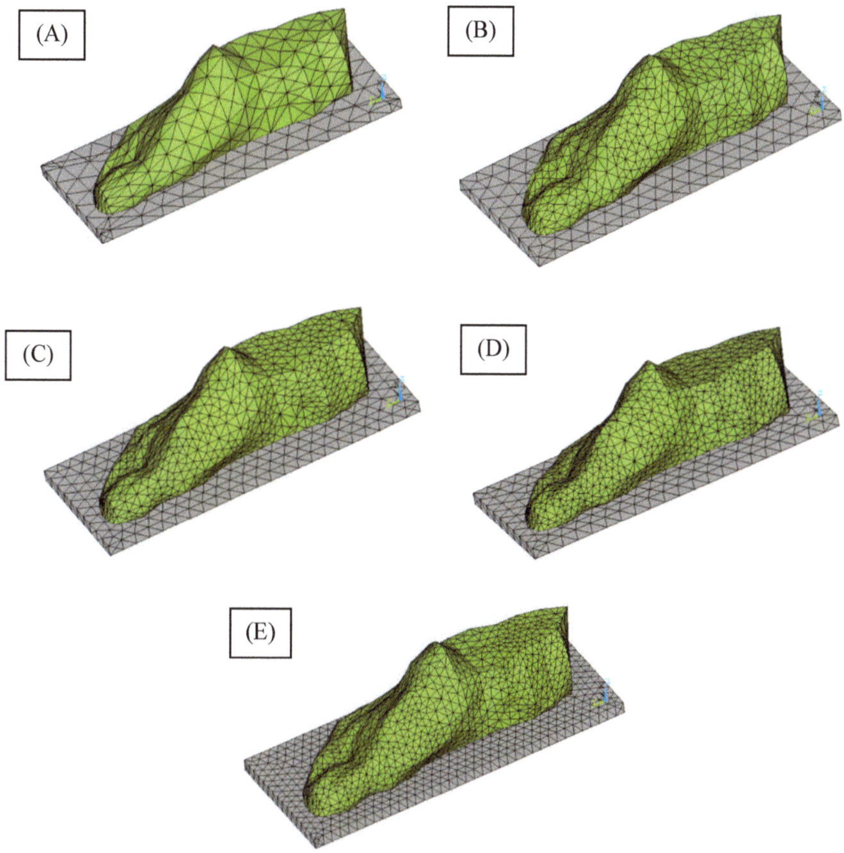

Fig. 3.6 Flat foot model and ground meshes: **a** Very coarse, **b** Coarse, **c** Semi-fine, **d** Fine, and **e** Very fine

precise simulation of foot dynamics. Additionally, we configured the surface-to-surface contact element to be bonded, accommodating initial penetration to better reflect actual conditions experienced during foot–ground interaction. To improve the accuracy of our surface contact representation and minimize unwanted penetration and gap closure during simulations, we implemented an automatic contact adjustment mechanism. This mechanism applied an initial contact closure factor of five to both the foot and ground models. By doing so, we ensured that interactions between the two surfaces were accurately captured and represented throughout the simulation process. This level of detail enhances the overall fidelity of the results obtained from this study, making our findings more relevant and impactful in the context of foot biomechanics and related applications.

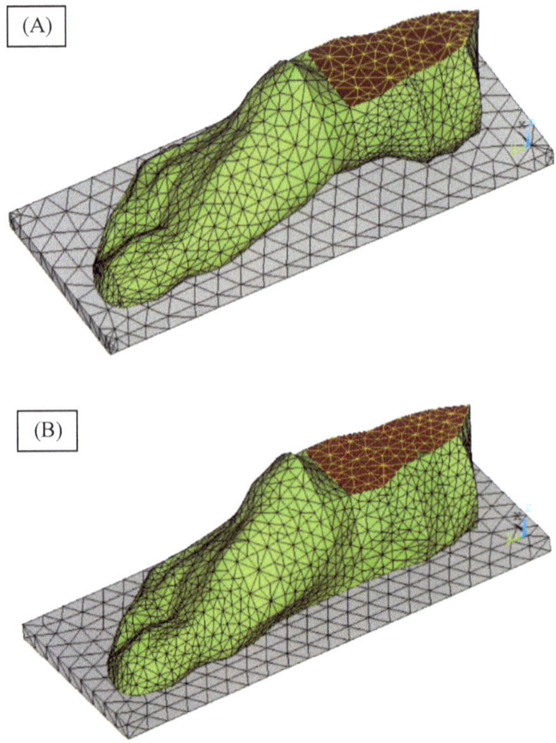

Fig. 3.7 Pressure load applied to the meshed model: **a** Normal foot and **b** Flatfoot. *Reproduced with permission from Elsevier* [19]

3.2.4 Material Modeling

The human foot is an intricate and multifaceted structure composed of numerous essential components that work together to facilitate movement, balance, and weight-bearing. One of the primary elements is the phalanges, which are the bones of the toes, categorized into three sections: distal, middle, and proximal. These bones are interconnected by interphalangeal joints, allowing for the flexibility and movement of the toes. In addition to the phalanges, the foot includes the metatarsal bones, which form the midsection and are crucial for distributing weight across the foot during activities such as walking and running. The metatarsophalangeal joints connect the toes to the metatarsals, playing an important role in toe function and support. Other notable components of the foot include the cuboid bone, which is located on the lateral side and aids in foot stability, and the calcaneus (heel bone), which is the largest bone in the foot and serves as a crucial point of contact with the ground. The talus bone, situated above the calcaneus, allows for the ankle's range of motion and connects the foot to the lower leg. The foot's structural complexity is further reinforced by its transition to the tibia and fibula, the two lengthy bones of the lower leg that support the foot's alignment and movement. In the field of biomechanics, extensive research has been conducted to develop detailed models that simulate the foot's

Table 3.1 Material properties for simulating the diabetic foot condition. *Reproduced with permission from Elsevier* [19]

Linear elastic parameters	Modulus of elasticity (MPa)	Poisson's ratio
Diabetic foot model	483	0.4
Ground	1e5	0.2

behavior under various environmental and mechanical conditions. These models are instrumental in studying how weight and pressure are distributed across both bony structures and the plantar surface, which is the area of the foot that makes contact with the ground. The current study specifically aims to investigate the effects of diabetic ulcers on the plantar surfaces of both flatfoot and normal foot presentations. This research is vital as it examines how mechanical stress is distributed at the sites of these ulcers, with the intention of identifying potential risks and implications for foot health in diabetic patients. To conduct this study, a simplified foot model was developed, accurately reflecting the typical geometric configuration and material properties of both bones and soft tissues associated with a diabetic foot condition. Values derived from existing literature were utilized to represent the elastic modulus and Poisson's ratio specific to the diabetic condition, emphasizing their importance in understanding how the foot reacts to mechanical stressors. Additionally, standard material values were incorporated to represent different ground surfaces, including hard surfaces like concrete and softer, flat ground conditions. These conditions are comprehensively outlined in Table 3.1. This thorough approach not only enhances our understanding of the mechanical consequences of diabetic ulcers but also has the potential to inform future treatment strategies aimed at improving outcomes for individuals affected by diabetes.

3.3 Results

This study conducted a comprehensive examination of the effects of DFUs on plantar stress distribution, focusing on a range of ulcer characteristics such as their unique locations, varying sizes, and differing depths. By analyzing these factors in detail, the research aimed to elucidate how each characteristic contributes to altered stress patterns within the foot. Additionally, the study made a comparative assessment of ulcerations in individuals with flat foot versus those with normal arches, ensuring that both groups were observed under identical conditions. This comparison highlighted significant differences in the patterns of stress distribution between the two foot types, revealing critical insights into how foot structure can influence the severity and implications of DFUs for treatment strategies. The subsequent sections of the study will delve into the findings, offering an in-depth discussion on how DFUs impact foot biomechanics. This exploration will include potential effects on gait, weight-bearing patterns, and overall foot health, emphasizing the importance of tailored treatment plans that consider the specific characteristics of both the ulcers and the individual's foot type.

3.3.1 Mesh Convergence Results

For standing loads of 0.1 MPa, 0.2 MPa, and 0.3 MPa, a comprehensive analysis was conducted to compare the maximum von Mises stress distribution between the normal foot and flat foot mesh models. In the case of the normal foot model, the analysis demonstrated a significant increase in the maximum von Mises stress as the mesh transitioned from a coarse configuration, which contained 2,645 elements, to a fine configuration with 11,144 elements. This increase in stress readings was consistently observed across all three applied load levels (as shown in Fig. 3.8a), indicating that the finer mesh improved the resolution of the stress distribution. Furthermore, when the analysis was extended to a superfine mesh containing 25,784 elements, it was found that the variations in peak von Mises stresses were minimal, remaining below 5%. This observation suggests that while the superfine mesh could provide additional detail, it did not significantly enhance the accuracy of the stress predictions when compared to the fine mesh. Consequently, the fine mesh with 11,144 elements was identified as optimal for subsequent analyses of the normal foot model, striking a balance between computational efficiency and the reliability of results. In parallel, a mesh convergence study was performed for the flat foot model. This analysis identified that the fine mesh configuration with 15,962 elements yielded the most accurate representation of stress distribution under the specified loading conditions. This selection was pivotal, as it ensured that the simulations would provide meaningful and reliable data regarding the mechanical behavior of flat foot structures as they responded to various loads (refer to Fig. 3.8b). By choosing this optimal mesh, the study lays a solid foundation for future investigations aimed at understanding the complexities of flat foot mechanics in greater detail.

3.3.2 Normal Foot

Without and with Ulcers

The stress distribution patterns within the plantar region of a normal diabetic foot are thoroughly illustrated in Fig. 3.9. This figure not only depicts an ulcer-free foot but also highlights various common ulcer sites, offering valuable insights into the biomechanical behavior of the foot under different conditions. To facilitate a meaningful comparison, a consistent ulcer size was employed in this analysis, with a diameter of 16 mm and a depth of 5 mm. This standardization ensures that the results drawn from comparing ulcerated and non-ulcerated states are both relevant and reliable. The analysis revealed that the stress distributions at the forefoot ulcer sites, specifically

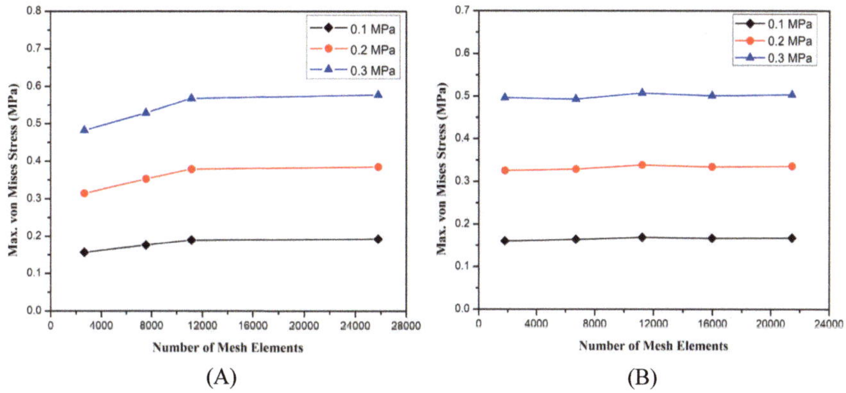

Fig. 3.8 Mesh convergence results for meshes: **a** Normal foot and **b** Flatfoot. *Reproduced with permission from Elsevier* [19]

at the hallux (big toe) and the first metatarsal, were largely uniform across the tested conditions, as evident in Fig. 3.9b and c. Notably, the stress patterns in these regions exhibited minimal variations when contrasted with the model representing a healthy foot devoid of ulcers, depicted in Fig. 3.9a. Remarkably, the maximum von Mises stress recorded at both the hallux and first metatarsal was measured at 0.568 MPa. This value is strikingly close to the stress levels observed in the ulcer-free model, indicating potential implications for clinical practice. This observation suggests that, for diabetic patients maintaining a standing position, there is no significant build-up of stress at these particular forefoot ulcer sites. This finding could influence how clinicians approach pressure management and ulcer prevention strategies for diabetic patients, ultimately guiding the development of targeted therapeutic measures.

The ulcer located at the lateral midfoot (refer to Fig. 3.6d) exhibited a notably elevated maximum stress level of 0.938 MPa, which translates to a significant 65% increase compared to the non-ulcer foot model, where the stress measurement was recorded at just 0.325 MPa. This observation suggests a significant shift in the distribution of maximum stress from the heel region to the midfoot corner, illuminating the profound effects of ulceration on pressure dynamics within the foot. In addition to the midfoot, substantial stress values were also identified in ulcer sites at both the medial and lateral heel regions. Specifically, the highest stress recorded at the medial heel (illustrated in Fig. 3.9e) was 0.800 MPa, while the lateral heel (shown in Fig. 3.9f) displayed a maximum stress of 0.888 MPa. These findings further underscore the urgent need for diligent monitoring and management of pressure distribution in diabetic patients. Increased stress at certain ulcer locations can hinder the healing process and elevate the risk of additional complications, ultimately impacting patient outcomes. Therefore, adequate pressure-relief strategies and careful evaluation of foot biomechanics are critical in preventing ulcer recurrence and ensuring effective treatment.

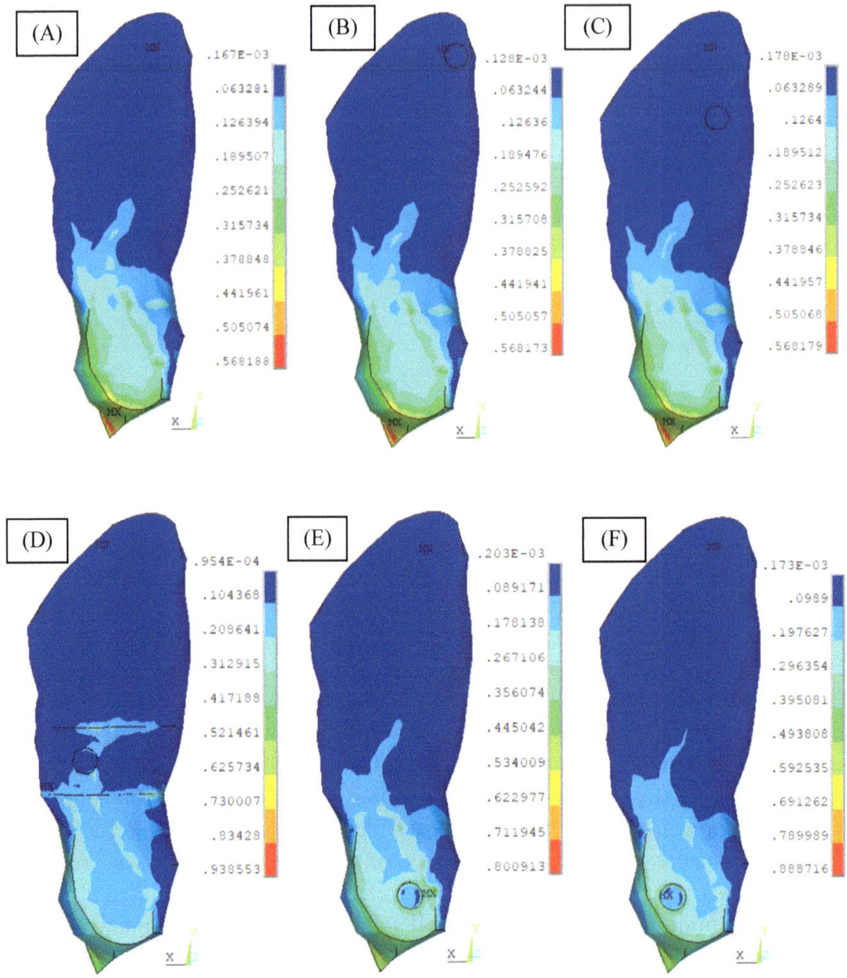

Fig. 3.9 Normal foot stresses for standing on hard ground: **a** Without ulcer, **b** Ulcer on hallux, **c** Ulcer on first metatarsal, **d** Ulcer on lateral midfoot, **e** Ulcer on medial heel, and **f** Ulcer on lateral heel. *Reproduced with permission from Elsevier* [19]

Effect of Ulcer Size and Depth

To achieve a precise simulation of various ulcer sites on the foot (as illustrated in Fig. 3.4), we designed foot models that incorporated two different ulcer sizes, 10 mm and 16 mm, and two distinct depths, 5 mm and 8 mm. This thorough approach enabled the development of a total of twenty unique models, calculated based on the combination of five anatomical sites, two sizes, and two depths (5 sites × 2 sizes × 2 depths). In Fig. 3.10, we present a detailed comparative analysis of the maximum von Mises stress observed across these models. This analysis provides insights into the stress distribution patterns at each ulcer site, highlighting how different parameters interact.

Notably, our data reveals that at the hallux (the big toe) and first metatarsal sites, variations in ulcer size and depth did not significantly impact stress concentration levels. Both sites consistently demonstrated a peak stress value of approximately 0.568 MPa, regardless of the modifications made to ulcer characteristics. This consistent finding suggests that the hallux and first metatarsal regions of the foot may exhibit a more uniform biomechanical response to changes in ulcer size and depth. Consequently, understanding this behavior could inform clinical approaches to ulcer management in these areas, emphasizing the need for targeted intervention strategies that account for the inherent mechanical stability of these sites. Overall, our research enhances the understanding of pressure distribution in foot ulcers and could pave the way for improved treatment protocols.

The lateral midfoot demonstrated a significantly broader range of von Mises stress values, fluctuating between 0.938 MPa and 0.972 MPa. This range indicates a pronounced sensitivity to both the size and depth of ulcers, which underscores the critical need for tailored interventions targeted at this particular area of the foot. When we investigated the effects of ulcer depth on stress concentration, we discovered that an increase in depth from 5 to 8 mm, while keeping the ulcer size constant, resulted in a negligible difference of less than 1% in the maximum stress value. This finding suggests that ulcer depth exerts only a minor influence on stress distribution for ulcers of this size. In contrast, when we modified the ulcer size from 10 to 16 mm while maintaining a constant depth, we observed a slightly more pronounced effect, with the maximum von Mises stress values varying by less than 2%. This indicates that size changes have a more substantial impact than depth modifications within

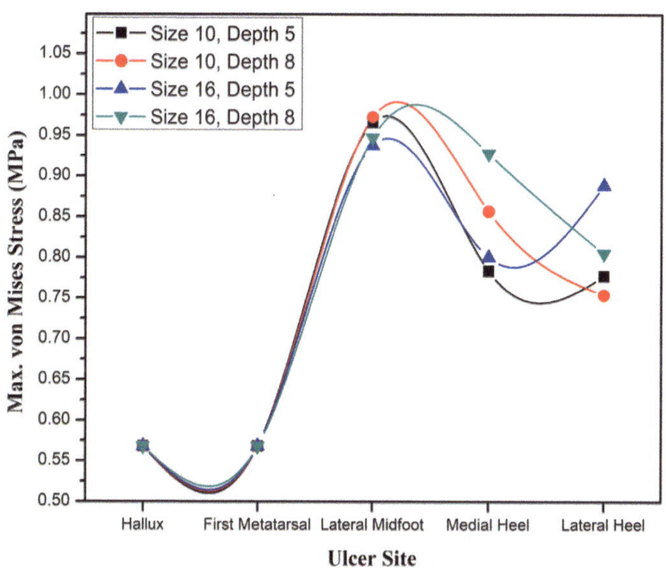

Fig. 3.10 Von Mises stress distribution for different ulcer sites on normal foot. The size and depth of the ulcer are in millimeters (mm). *Reproduced with permission from Elsevier* [19]

this range. An in-depth analysis of ulcer sites located on the heel revealed a more intricate relationship among size, depth, and stress concentration patterns. Focusing on the medial heel, we found that increasing the ulcer size from 10 to 16 mm at a consistent depth of 8 mm led to a significant 8% increase in stress concentration, escalating the maximum stress from 0.857 MPa to 0.928 MPa. Conversely, when the depth was reduced to 5 mm, the change in ulcer size had a minimal impact on the maximum stress observed, indicating that shallower depths may not be as sensitive to size variations. Moreover, we recorded considerable increases in maximum von Mises stress when the depth shifted from 5 to 8 mm, with a 10% increase noted for the 10 mm ulcer size and a more dramatic 16% increase for the 16 mm ulcer size. This highlights that although changes in size at a shallower depth have little effect, increasing depth plays a substantial role in amplifying stress levels for both sizes. Notably, at the lateral heel, we recorded the highest maximum von Mises stress of 0.888 MPa for an ulcer size of 16 mm at a depth of 5 mm. This remarkable finding emphasizes the importance of considering both the size and depth of ulcers when assessing stress distribution in foot ulcers. Both factors are crucially influential in understanding and managing the development of pressure ulcers, where tailored prevention and treatment strategies can greatly enhance patient outcomes.

3.3.3 Flat Foot

Without and with Ulcers

Figure 3.11 illustrates the distribution of von Mises stress across the plantar surfaces of flat foot, specifically comparing conditions with and without the presence of ulcers. In all models analyzed, the maximum von Mises stress, measured at the corner of the heel, was observed to be 0.501 MPa. This base measurement, while consistent across the models, exhibited notable variations in the context of lateral heel ulceration. When examining the stress distribution patterns in flat foot with ulcers located at various sites, including the hallux (Fig. 3.11b), first metatarsal (Fig. 3.11c), and medial heel (Fig. 3.11e), we found that these distributions closely mirrored those of the flat foot configuration without any ulcers (Fig. 3.11a). This similarity suggests that, in these particular cases, the presence of ulcers did not materially influence the mechanical stress distribution in those regions of the foot. Conversely, the lateral heel ulceration (Fig. 3.11f) demonstrated a striking increase in stress values, peaking at 0.714 MPa. This marked increase signifies a substantial 42.5% rise in stress compared to baseline measurements recorded from the same area in a flat foot without ulcerations. Such an elevated stress state is critical, as it underscores the potentially harmful impact of ulceration on foot mechanics, particularly in the lateral heel region. These findings highlight the need for targeted and effective interventions for individuals with flat foot and corresponding ulcerations. By understanding the distinct patterns of mechanical stress, healthcare providers can develop tailored treatment strategies that address the specific challenges posed by ulcerations, ultimately improving the quality of life and mobility for those affected.

Effect of Ulcer Size and Depth

Figure 3.12 illustrates an in-depth comparison of various combinations of ulcer locations, sizes, and depths specifically analyzed within the flat foot model. The analysis reveals that the maximum stress values for ulcers located in critical areas, such as the hallux, first metatarsal, lateral midfoot, and medial heel, were notably consistent, each recording approximately 0.501 MPa. This uniformity indicates that, despite differing ulcer characteristics, these regions likely experience similar mechanical loads, which may have implications for treatment strategies and risk assessments. In

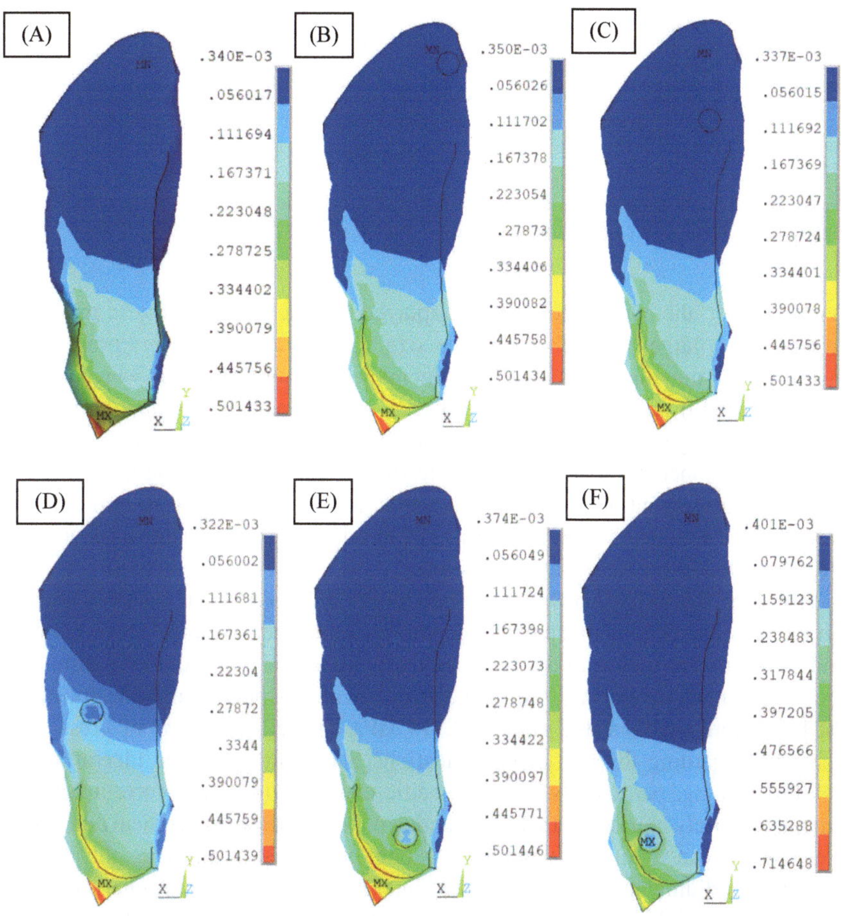

Fig. 3.11 Flat foot stresses for standing on hard ground: **a** Without ulcer, **b** Ulcer on hallux, **c** Ulcer on first metatarsal, **d** Ulcer on lateral midfoot, **e** Ulcer on medial heel, and **f** Ulcer on lateral heel. *Reproduced with permission from Elsevier* [19]

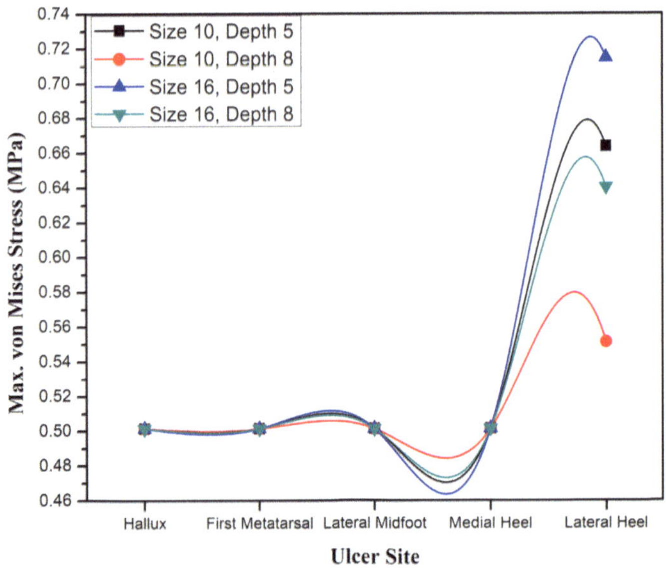

Fig. 3.12 Maximum von Mises stresses for different ulcer sites on the flat foot model. The size and depth of the ulcer are in millimeters (mm). *Reproduced with permission from Elsevier* [19]

stark contrast, the lateral heel region displayed significant variability in maximum stress values, largely influenced by the size and depth of the ulcers present. For instance, a 10 mm diameter ulcer in the lateral heel demonstrated that when its depth was increased from 5 to 8 mm, there was an approximate 17% reduction in stress levels. This suggests that as ulcers become deeper in this area, they may experience lower stress concentrations, potentially leading to improved healing outcomes and shaping management approaches for patients. Moreover, a larger 16 mm diameter ulcer in the same region showcased a similar trend, wherein increasing its depth from 5 to 8 mm led to a 10% reduction in stress.

However, this reduction was less pronounced compared to that observed with the smaller ulcer, indicating that the relationship between ulcer size and depth is complex and may vary from case to case. Notably, among all the configurations simulated, the largest ulcer, measuring 16 mm in diameter with a depth of 5 mm, demonstrated the highest maximum stress value of 0.714 MPa. This elevated level of stress raises concerns regarding the risk of complications, including increased ulceration and delayed healing, particularly in this specific configuration. Therefore, it becomes crucial to closely monitor both the size and depth of ulcers within clinical practice, as these factors can significantly influence patient outcomes. In summary, this detailed comparison illuminates the sophisticated interactions between ulcer characteristics, such as size and depth, and the resulting mechanical stresses they encounter in the flat foot model. Understanding these relationships is vital for developing effective preventive strategies and interventions in clinical settings.

3.4 Discussion

In a comprehensive series of simulations aimed at examining the biomechanical differences between a diabetic normal foot and flat foot, we conducted a detailed analysis of stress distribution within the plantar soft tissue at designated ulcer locations. These simulations were conducted to maintain consistency in ulcer size, depth, and site across both foot types, thereby ensuring the reliability of our results. As shown in Table 3.2, we recorded the mean values of maximum von Mises stress at five distinct ulcer sites, factoring in variations in ulcer sizes and depths. Our analysis revealed that the average maximum stress observed in the normal foot was significantly higher, measuring 0.748 MPa, in contrast to the 0.529 MPa recorded for the flat foot. This notable disparity in stress levels was consistent across all ulcer sites we examined, highlighting a fundamental difference in mechanical responses between the two foot types. Among the various ulcer sites evaluated, the lateral midfoot region demonstrated the highest mean stress in the normal foot model, peaking at 0.956 MPa. This was closely followed by the medial heel at 0.842 MPa and the lateral heel at 0.806 MPa. These findings suggest that the lateral midfoot is particularly susceptible to increased stress, a factor that could significantly contribute to the formation of ulcers in diabetic patients possessing a normal foot structure. In contrast, the flat foot model exhibited a different pattern of stress distribution; the lateral midfoot was the only ulcer site to record a slightly elevated mean maximum stress, at 0.642 MPa. This observation underscores the altered mechanical properties of the flat foot, which may influence the overall distribution of stress across the plantar soft tissue, possibly reducing the risk of ulcer formation at other sites while increasing vulnerability in specific areas. Overall, our study sheds light on the critical variations in stress distribution due to anatomical differences between normal and flat foot, emphasizing the need for tailored interventions to prevent ulcer formation in diabetic patients [25, 26].

In the evaluation of the normal foot model, researchers consistently observed similar maximum stress levels in the lateral midfoot region across a range of ulcer sizes and depths. This indicates that the stress distribution in this area is relatively uniform, regardless of the characteristics of the ulcers, suggesting that the normal anatomical structure of the foot effectively distributes stress without significant deviation. In contrast, the flat foot model exhibited a more complex pattern of stress distribution. Here, maximum stress levels varied across nearly all ulcer sites, with the notable exception of the lateral heel. This variation suggests that anatomical

Table 3.2 Mean values for the max. von mises stress distribution (MPa). *Reproduced with permission from Elsevier* [19]

Locations	Hallux	First metatarsal	Lateral midfoot	Medial heel	Lateral heel
Normal foot	0.568 ± 0	0.568 ± 0	0.956 ± 0.013	0.842 ± 0.055	0.806 ± 0.049
Flatfoot	0.501 ± 0	0.501 ± 0	0.501 ± 0	0.501 ± 0	0.642 ± 0.057

differences in the flat foot significantly influence how stress is distributed across the plantar surface. In the medial heel region, a significant finding emerged: maximum stress levels increased with greater ulcer depth for ulcers of the same size. This direct relationship implies that deeper ulcers could pose a greater risk for additional tissue damage, which may complicate healing. However, within the same group of ulcer depths in the medial heel, researchers did not find consistent trends in maximum stress levels. This lack of uniformity may indicate the presence of other influencing factors, such as the unique biomechanical properties associated with flat foot deformity, which can lead to unpredictable stress responses depending on individual variations in foot structure and function. In the lateral heel region, the findings were particularly distinctive. Here, the data showed that larger ulcer sizes, when combined with lower ulcer depths, resulted in increased maximum stress levels. This relationship highlights the intricate interplay between size and depth in determining how stress is experienced at this site. Notably, similar trends in stress distribution related to ulcer size and depth were also recorded at this ulcer site within the flat foot model, reinforcing the need for tailored assessment and treatment strategies that consider both the mechanical and anatomical factors at play in ulcer management.

Figure 3.13 provides a detailed illustration of the stress values measured at four distinct points on the ulcer site located on the lateral heel for both normal and flat foot models. In both cases, the peak stress was consistently observed in the bottom left corner of the ulcer site, which highlights this area as a significant concern for ulcer development. When analyzing the stress distributions, the normal foot model displayed a more uniform stress profile. The variation in stress values among the four measured points was less than 30%, indicating that the normal foot is more adept at distributing weight evenly. This uniformity suggests that individuals with a normal foot structure may experience a lower risk of localized pressure, making their foot more resilient to uneven stress distribution during activities such as walking or standing. In contrast, the flat foot model revealed considerable disparities in stress distribution, particularly on the left wall of the ulcer. Here, the stress values were found to be over twice as high compared to those on the right wall, illustrating a stark imbalance. This pronounced difference in stress distribution poses a higher risk for the ulcer to expand laterally, especially towards the left wall. Such expansion could complicate the healing process and necessitate targeted interventions, such as customized orthotics or specific therapeutic strategies aimed at redistributing pressure. Overall, these findings underscore the critical importance of considering foot morphology, such as the structural differences between normal and flat foot, when assessing ulcer dynamics.

3.5 Conclusions

This study aimed to comprehensively investigate the biomechanics of DFUs through the use of biofidelic computational modeling. We developed a detailed full-scale foot model to accurately simulate common ulcer locations, sizes, and depths, specifically

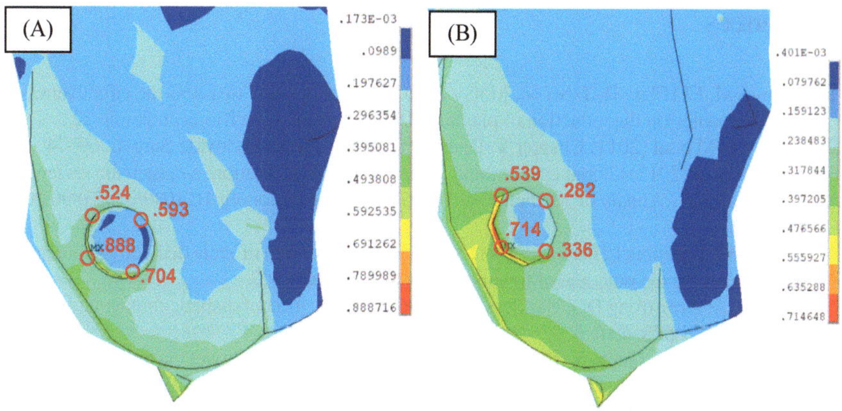

Fig. 3.13 Stress at the lateral heel ulcer: **a** Normal foot and **b** Flat foot. *Reproduced with permission from Elsevier* [19]

focusing on both normal and flat feet. When the foot model was subjected to standing loads, it was discovered that the maximum stress experienced in the plantar region was similar for forefoot ulcers in both types of foot, indicating a shared response to pressure in the forefoot area. However, the analysis revealed that the normal foot exhibited significantly higher maximum stresses in the midfoot and heel regions compared to the flat foot. In the case of the flat foot, significant increases in maximum stress were observed primarily in the lateral heel region, where ulcers are particularly prevalent. These findings align with existing medical knowledge, highlighting the higher incidence of diabetic ulcers in the heel area, which is often subjected to more pressure and less cushioning [27–29]. Additionally, the study revealed that the geometry of the ulcer itself had a substantial impact on stress distribution, especially in the heel of the normal foot and even more markedly in the lateral heel of the flat foot. Specifically, larger ulcers with lower depths in the heel region were found to generate maximum stress, which raises concerns about their susceptibility to worsening conditions. The lateral heel ulcer in a flat foot exhibited a nonuniform stress distribution along its wall, suggesting that this particular area may require careful monitoring and intervention to prevent further complications or the development of additional ulcers. Overall, this detailed investigation into the biomechanics of DFUs provides critical insights that can enhance the understanding and management of this condition. The findings will serve as valuable guidelines for healthcare professionals, including doctors and surgeons, in their efforts to prevent and treat DFUs effectively. By addressing these biomechanics, healthcare providers can improve patient care and outcomes for those at risk of developing diabetic ulcers.

References

1. Ibrahim M, El Hilaly R, Taher M, Morsy A (2013) A pilot study to assess the effectiveness of orthotic insoles on the reduction of plantar soft tissue strain. Clin Biomech 28:68–72
2. Lepäntalo M et al (2011) Chapter V: Diabetic foot. Eur J Vasc Endovasc Surg 42:60–74
3. Zhang P et al (2017) Global epidemiology of diabetic foot ulceration: a systematic review and meta-analysis†. Annals of Medicine 49 106–116. at https://doi.org/10.1080/07853890.2016.1231932
4. Kaufman J, Breeding L, Rosenberg N (1987) Anatomic location of acute diabetic foot infection: Its influence on the outcome of treatment. Am Surg 53:109–112
5. Lavery LA, Armstrong DG, Harkless LB (1996) Classification of diabetic foot wounds. J Foot Ankle Surg 35:528–531
6. Bose D, Singh G, Gupta S, Chanda A (2024) Development of a novel customized insole for effective pressure offloading in diabetic patients. Prosthes. 6, Pages 341–356
7. Gupta S et al (2023) Diabot: development of a diabetic foot pressure tracking device. J 6, Pages 32–47
8. Chhikara K, Singh G, Gupta S, Chanda A (2022) Progress of additive manufacturing in fabrication of foot orthoses for diabetic patients: A review. Ann 3D Print Med 8, 100085
9. Oyibo SO et al (2001) The effects of ulcer size and site, patient's age, sex and type and duration of diabetes on the outcome of diabetic foot ulcers. Diabet Med 18:133–138
10. Lemmon D, Shiang TY, Hashmi A, Ulbrecht JS, Cavanagh PR (1997) The effect of insoles in therapeutic footwear—A finite element approach. J Biomech 30:615–620
11. Caputo GM, Cavanagh PR, Ulbrecht JS, Gibbons GW, Karchmer AW (1994) Assessment and management of foot disease in patients with diabetes. N Engl J Med 331:854–860
12. Turner DE, Helliwell PS, Burton AK, Woodburn J (2007) The relationship between passive range of motion and range of motion during gait and plantar pressure measurements. Diabet Med 24:1240–1246
13. Singh G, Chanda A (2024) Finite element modeling of diabetic foot: a state-of-the-art review. Eng Res Express 6:012507
14. Gupta S, Singh G, Chanda A (2021) Prediction of diabetic foot ulcer progression: a computational study. Biomed Phys Eng Express 7:065020
15. Pourghasem M, Kamali N, Farsi M, Soltanpour N (2016) Prevalence of flatfoot among school students and its relationship with BMI. Acta Orthop Traumatol Turc 50:554–557
16. Filardi V (2018) Flatfoot and normal foot a comparative analysis of the stress shielding. J Orthop 15:820–825
17. Telfer S, Erdemir A, Woodburn J, Cavanagh PR (2014) What has finite element analysis taught us about diabetic foot disease and its management? A Systematic Review. PLoS One 9:e109994
18. Chanda A, Unnikrishnan V (2018) Novel insole design for diabetic foot ulcer management. Proc Inst Mech Eng Part H J Eng Med. 232, 1182–1195
19. Singh G, Gupta S, Chanda A (2021) Biomechanical modelling of diabetic foot ulcers: A computational study. J Biomech 127:110699
20. Mishra SC, Chhatbar KC, Kashikar A, Mehndiratta A (2017) Diabetic foot. BMJ 359:j5064
21. Barani Z, Haghpanahi M, Katoozian H (2005) Three dimensional stress analysis of diabetic insole: A finite element approach. Technol Heal Care 13:185–192
22. Frykberg RG (2002) Diabetic foot ulcers: pathogenesis and management. American Family Physician 66
23. Besse JL, Leemrijse T, Deleu PA (2011) Diabetic foot: The orthopedic surgery angle. Orthop Traumatol: Surg Res 97 314–329 at https://doi.org/10.1016/j.otsr.2011.03.001
24. Singh G, Chanda A (2022) Biomechanical modeling of progressive wound healing: A computational study. Biomed Eng Adv 4:100055
25. Singh G, Bose D, Chanda A (2025) Development and testing of a novel diabetic orthosis for plantar pressure reduction. Facta Univ Ser Mech Eng. https://doi.org/10.22190/FUME240725044S

26. Singh G, Lamba A, Chanda A (2024) Role of additive manufacturing for the management of diabetic foot ulcers. In Addit Manuf Biomed Appl 19–38 (Springer, Singapore). https://doi.org/10.1007/978-981-97-5456-4_2
27. Putti AB, Arnold GP, Cochrane L, Abboud RJ (2007) The Pedar® in-shoe system: Repeatability and normal pressure values. Gait Posture 25:401–405
28. Bus SA, Ulbrecht JS, Cavanagh PR (2004) Pressure relief and load redistribution by custom-made insoles in diabetic patients with neuropathy and foot deformity. Clin Biomech 19:629–638
29. Cavanagh PR, Rodgers MM, Liboshi A (1987) Pressure distribution under symptom-free feet during barefoot standing. Foot Ankle Int 7:262–278

Chapter 4
Computational Modeling of Diabetic Ulcers Across All Possible Locations

4.1 Introduction

Foot ulcers represent a serious, expensive, and prevalent complication associated with diabetes. These ulcers not only disrupt a person's ability to move but can also deteriorate over time or lead to the formation of additional ulcers when healing does not proceed normally in diabetic individuals [1–4]. In severe cases, untreated foot ulcers may necessitate amputations, significantly impacting the patient's quality of life. Diabetic patients with foot ulcers typically exhibit higher plantar pressures compared to individuals with healthy foot [5–7]. This increased pressure can result from uneven distribution of weight during walking, leading to irregular foot loading, which creates stress concentrations in certain areas. These mechanical stresses heighten the risk of new ulcerations forming [8, 9]. Studies conducted by researchers such as Kogani et al. and Jeong et al. have indicated that reducing plantar pressure by at least 30% can be crucial in preventing foot ulcers among diabetic patients [10–12]. Custom insoles and therapeutic shoes have been identified as effective tools for achieving this reduction, as they can help distribute pressure more evenly across the foot. Furthermore, clinical studies have found that factors such as the location, depth, and size of an ulcer can significantly influence its progression and healing. Most foot ulcers in diabetic patients are observed on the plantar region, particularly at the forefoot and heel; however, it is also common for ulcers to develop in the midfoot area due to excessive loading [13, 14]. Diabetic foot ulcers (DFUs) pose numerous challenges, primarily due to the intricate nature of accurately measuring foot loading. Additionally, there are biosafety and ethical issues to consider when experimenting with diabetic populations, making it difficult to establish comprehensive guidelines for prevention and treatment [15, 16]. Addressing these challenges through innovative research methodologies is essential for better understanding and managing DFUs, ultimately improving outcomes for affected individuals [17, 18].

Recently, computational modeling has emerged as a valuable tool for examining the complexities of DFUs following ulceration [4, 19–21]. In a study conducted

A. Chanda and G. Singh, *Diabetic Foot Ulcer*, Biomedical Materials for Multi-functional Applications, https://doi.org/10.1007/978-981-95-2484-6_4

by Chanda et al. [22], they explored how different activities, such as standing and walking, influence the plantar pressures experienced in a diabetic foot model that included both regularly shaped and irregularly shaped ulcers. Their simulations focused on two common ulcer locations: the toe and the heel. The researchers estimated the wall stresses surrounding these ulcers, revealing some concerning findings. Specifically, they noted that the stresses along the walls of heel ulcers were significantly higher than normal, indicating a substantial risk for further ulcer growth in these areas. This finding underscores the importance of monitoring heel ulcers closely, as the increased pressure could exacerbate the condition. Moreover, the study recorded elevated stresses at various other locations on the foot, which raises the potential for developing new ulcers in these areas. This highlights the broader implications for diabetic foot care, suggesting that different regions of the foot are at risk due to altered pressures during common activities. Understanding these dynamics through computational modeling could inform better preventive strategies and treatments for individuals with DFUs [23–25].

In this study, we developed a comprehensive full-scale model of the human foot to explore the mechanical stresses associated with various locations of ulcers, particularly in individuals with diabetes. Our objective was not only to understand existing ulcer sites but also to predict new potential ulceration sites that may occur due to elevated plantar stress concentrations. To achieve this, we simulated a total of 52 distinct ulcer locations, each examined in isolation. The simulations accounted for the varying loads that the foot experiences during common activities such as standing and walking. By normalizing the stresses generated in these simulations according to the foot size, we ensured consistent results that facilitate direct comparisons across different ulcer locations. The collected data underwent rigorous statistical analysis, allowing us to derive innovative formulations aimed at predicting peak plantar stresses. These formulations serve a dual purpose: they not only forecast the stresses experienced at known ulcer sites but also help pinpoint other specific areas on the foot that may be at increased risk for developing new ulcers under similar stress conditions. Our research significantly deepens the understanding of diabetic foot mechanics, providing valuable insights into the dynamics of foot health. These findings have practical implications for clinical assessments of foot conditions and emphasize the importance of preventative measures in managing pressure-related injuries among diabetic patients. By identifying stress concentrations and potential ulceration sites, healthcare professionals can better tailor interventions to mitigate the risks associated with diabetic foot complications.

4.2 Materials and Methods

4.2.1 Geometrical Modeling

To develop a comprehensive foot model for this study, we marked a total of 301 points on the right foot of a human subject who was seated comfortably in a chair. The first step involved defining a reference framework by establishing an origin point, from which we accurately recorded the X, Y, and Z coordinates of each marked point using three precise movable rulers. This method ensured that we captured accurate measurements while the foot remained stationary throughout the process. To enhance the reliability of our measurements, we established multiple fixed reference points: three located on the midfoot, two on the heel, and one on the forefoot. These reference points were regularly monitored during the data collection phase to confirm that the foot maintained its position. Any potential movement could introduce errors that would compromise the measurement integrity, so this precaution was essential. Once the coordinates were accurately recorded, we utilized Ansys APDL 2019 R2 to plot the data in three-dimensional space. This plotting allowed us to visualize the foot's structure in detail. We then created a wire mesh by connecting the marked points with splines, resulting in a comprehensive representation of the foot (refer to Fig. 4.1a). Following this, we selected sets of four adjacent lines to form small surface areas, which were interconnected to create a solid foot volume comprising 16 distinct subvolumes (refer to Fig. 4.1b). The modeling methodology employed in this study was designed to enhance control over the meshing process of the discretized volumes. This approach was essential for the subsequent simulations of ulcers, ensuring a high-quality mesh that would provide consistent results, irrespective of any variations in mesh sizing. The primary aim of this investigation was to analyze how ulcers, often a concern for diabetic patients, affect plantar stresses within the foot. Given this focus, the solid foot model was considered optimal for addressing such inquiries. To further improve the realism of our testing scenarios, we also modeled a ground surface beneath the foot, applying a thickness of 10 mm. This realistic setting was crucial for accurately simulating the conditions under which plantar stresses occur (see Fig. 4.1b). By creating this detailed foot model, we aimed to enhance our understanding of how ulcer development impacts foot dynamics, ultimately contributing to improved clinical practices and patient care.

DFUs can vary widely in size, ranging from just 1 mm to as large as 70 mm. This variation significantly impacts the severity of the ulcers and their associated healing outcomes. Research indicates that ulcers measuring less than 10 mm tend to have an exceptional healing rate of 100%, which underscores the importance of early intervention [27, 28]. Conversely, ulcers that exceed 50 mm present a much more challenging clinical scenario; approximately 73% of patients with these larger ulcers may require minor amputations due to complications associated with their condition, highlighting the urgency of addressing these larger wounds promptly [20]. In this study, the primary focus is on simulating nonhealing ulcers, specifically using circular models with a diameter of 16 mm and a depth of 5 mm. This choice of dimensions

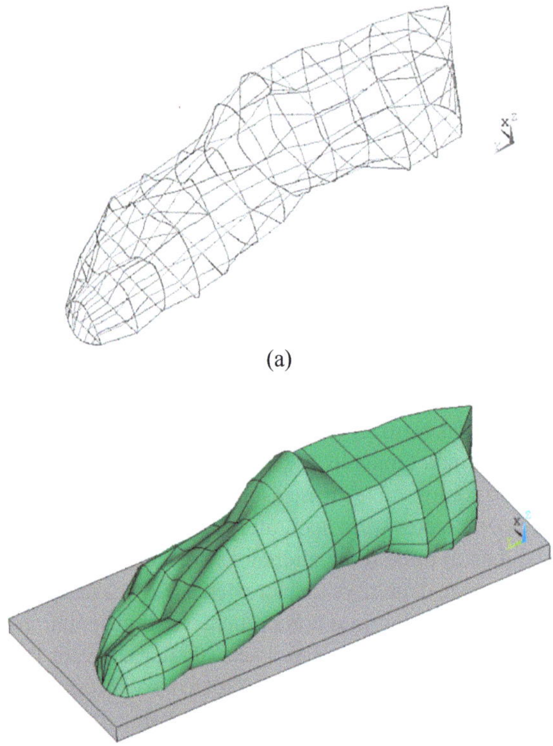

(a)

(b)

Fig. 4.1 **a** Line wire mesh created by connecting the measured foot coordinates and **b** Foot and ground volumes. *Reproduced with permission from IOP Science* [26]

is based on prevalent clinical presentations, making it a relevant and realistic model [29, 30]. By studying ulcers of this size and shape, researchers can gain valuable insights into the behavior of nonhealing ulcers, investigate their responses to various treatment options, and develop strategies to improve healing outcomes for patients with diabetic foot complications.

To conduct a thorough analysis of ulcer locations on the foot, we designated the topmost right area of the plantar region as the origin point for our coordinate system. This strategic choice allows for consistent referencing across various cases. We subsequently developed a specialized nomenclature for the coordinates that correspond to potential ulcer sites, ensuring clarity and precision in our findings. The X coordinates, which represent the width of the foot, were normalized to a standard foot width of 99 mm. Similarly, the Y coordinates, which indicate the length of the foot, were normalized to a standard length of 254 mm. The process of normalization is vital because it allows us to apply the study's findings universally, despite the inherent variability in foot geometry among different individuals. This variability can stem from factors such as genetics, age, and activity levels, which significantly influence foot shape and size. The rationale behind this normalization is rooted in the necessity for standardized foot size measurements, which play a crucial role in various industries, including footwear manufacturing and orthotic design. Adhering to these standards, as specified in ISO standard ISO 9407:2019, ensures that the results of our study can be reliably used in practical applications. While acknowledging that this approach may not fully capture every individual's unique foot dimension, it serves as a robust framework for extrapolating our findings to a wider population. This method sets a solid foundation for further research and improvements in ulcer prevention and treatment strategies, ultimately benefiting individuals at risk of foot ulcers.

A comprehensive analysis of ulcer locations has resulted in the identification of 52 distinct sites on the plantar surface of the foot. To achieve this mapping, 11 precise points were marked along the X-axis and 16 corresponding points on the Y-axis. These points were systematically selected to maintain approximately equal distance intervals, ensuring a thorough and balanced assessment of ulcer distribution across the surface. Specifically, the ulcer locations on the Y-axis were designated at the following coordinates: 0.1063L, 0.1732L, 0.2402L, 0.3071L, 0.3740L, 0.4409L, 0.5079L, 0.5748L, 0.6417L, 0.7087L, 0.7756L, 0.8425L, 0.9094L, and 0.9567L, as illustrated in Fig. 4.2a. This careful selection of points provides a clear framework for understanding how ulcer development can vary along the vertical axis of the foot. In a similar fashion, the ulcer locations along the X-axis were established at the following coordinates: 0.1460W, 0.2015W, 0.2268W, 0.3177W, 0.3985W, 0.4894W, 0.5702W, 0.6611W, and 0.8328W, as shown in Fig. 4.2b. Mapping these coordinates allows for a detailed examination of where ulcers are most likely to arise on the horizontal plane. Such precise mapping not only enhances our understanding of ulcer distribution but also provides critical insights for clinical practices related to diabetic foot care. By identifying these specific locations, healthcare professionals can better assess patients' risk factors, develop preventative strategies, and improve overall patient outcomes in managing diabetic foot health.

4.2.2 Material Properties

The human foot is a remarkably intricate structure consisting of 26 bones, which include the talus, calcaneus, tarsals, metatarsals, phalanges, and sesamoids. This skeletal framework provides both support and mobility, allowing for a wide range of movements essential for activities such as walking, running, and jumping. Supporting this bony architecture is a complex network of muscles, tendons, and ligaments. Key components include the plantar fascia, which helps maintain the arch of the foot; the plantar calcaneonavicular ligament, also known as the spring ligament, which supports the arch during weight-bearing activities; and the calcaneocuboid ligament, which contributes to the stability of the foot's lateral aspect. Together, these structures play crucial roles in providing stability, shock absorption, and mobility. Extensive research in biomechanics has led to the development of detailed foot models that analyze various aspects of foot function, including loading patterns during different activities and the effects of stress shielding. This research is particularly relevant in the context of the diabetic foot. Studies have shown that diabetic ulcers can significantly

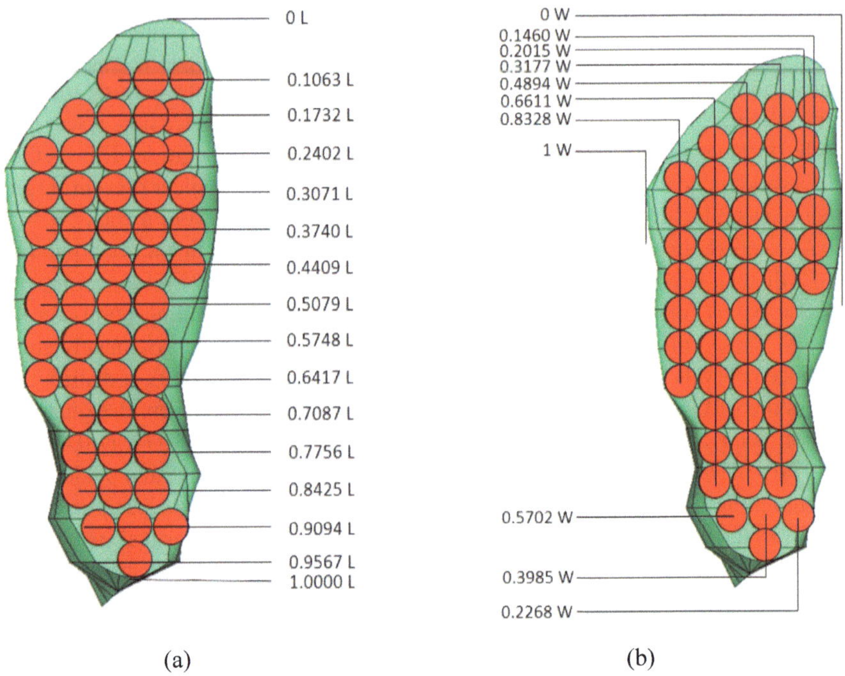

Fig. 4.2 52 Ulcer locations marked along: **a** Length (Y axis) and **b** Width (Y axis). *Reproduced with permission from IOP Science* [26]

alter the distribution of plantar stress, potentially leading to further complications, progression of the ulcers, or recurrence even after healing. To enhance understanding of these processes, vital parameters such as the modulus of elasticity and Poisson's ratio have been derived from existing literature to inform computational models [22]. The values selected in Table 4.1 represent optimal material properties for a diabetic foot, taking into account factors such as standing loads and an average of the geometric configurations and material characteristics of the affected bones and soft tissues. By integrating these insights, researchers aim to improve prevention strategies and treatment options for individuals at risk of foot complications due to diabetes.

Table 4.1 Material properties simulating the diabetic foot. *Reproduced with permission from IOP Science* [26]

Material model	Modulus of elasticity (MPa)	Poisson's ratio
Diabetic foot model	483	0.4
Ground	1E5	0.2

4.2.3 Finite Element Modeling

The finite element (FE) analysis was conducted using Ansys APDL 2019R2, a software tool widely used in engineering simulations. The geometries involved in the study were carefully meshed using 20-node solid tetrahedral elements known as Solid 186. This particular element type was specifically chosen for its ability to effectively model large deformations and complex contact interactions, both of which are crucial for accurately analyzing biological structures [31–33]. For instance, when examining the foot, it is essential to account for the intricate responses to load variations and movement, as well as the interactions between different anatomical components. The use of these advanced elements ensures that the simulation results are reliable and can provide valuable insights into the mechanical behavior of such complex biological systems [34, 35].

A detailed mesh convergence study was undertaken to thoroughly investigate the influence of various mesh configurations on the accuracy of simulation results. This study analyzed five distinct mesh types, which are visually represented in Fig. 4.3. The configurations evaluated included a very coarse mesh comprised of 4,726 elements, a coarse mesh with 10,249 elements, a fine mesh containing 16,699 elements, a very fine mesh with 21,916 elements, and the finest mesh model featuring 27,834 elements. To accurately simulate realistic standing and walking loads, three specific pressure values were employed throughout the mesh convergence study: 0.1 MPa, 0.2 MPa, and 0.3 MPa [22]. It is essential to highlight that for all simulations conducted, the maximum foot pressure load of 0.3 MPa was specifically applied to the optimal mesh configuration identified during the convergence study. This peak pressure value was distributed across the contact surface of the foot to replicate real-life loading scenarios as closely as possible. By simulating the pressure distribution in this way, the study aimed to provide realistic insight into the foot's behavior under different loading conditions, which is crucial for understanding foot–ground interactions. These details are further illustrated in Fig. 4.3b, which showcases the distribution pattern of the pressure across the foot's surface, emphasizing the significance of the chosen mesh configuration in achieving accurate simulation outcomes.

In order to establish appropriate boundary conditions for the simulation, the bottom surface of the ground was fixed in all degrees of freedom. This measure was essential to prevent any movement during the simulations, ensuring that the results would accurately reflect realistic conditions. To effectively capture the complex interaction between the foot and the ground, a flexible contact pair was developed. This contact pair featured a penetration tolerance set to 0.15, which permitted slight interpenetration during moments of contact. This allowance is crucial, as it closely mirrors the natural deformation that occurs when a foot makes contact with various surfaces. Additionally, a penalty stiffness value of 0.25 was implemented to control the force response during these contact interactions. This parameter determines how quickly and forcefully the system responds to interpenetration, thus influencing the overall behavior during simulations. These specific parameters were chosen with great care to ensure a comprehensive and realistic transfer of loads, accurately representing

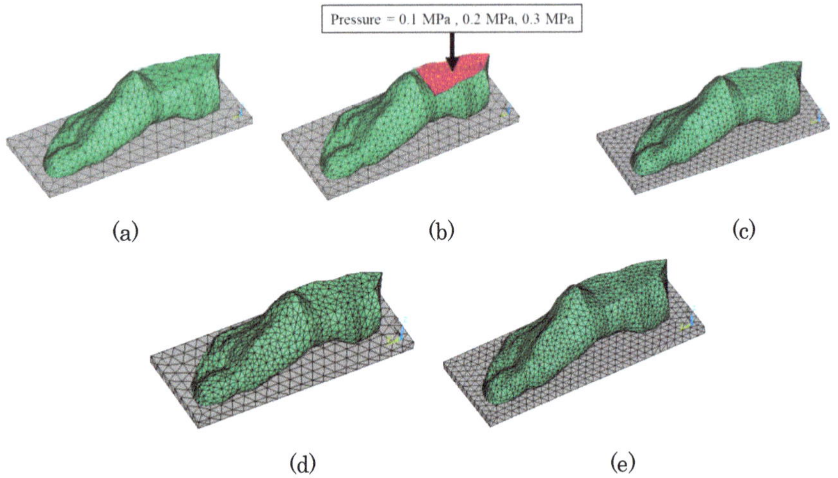

Fig. 4.3 Foot model and ground meshes used in mesh convergence study, and the loading applied: **a** Very coarse, **b** Coarse, **c** Fine, **d** Very fine, and **e** Finest. *Reproduced with permission from IOP Science* [26]

the intricate dynamics of foot–ground interactions. This includes not only the static conditions present while standing but also the varying conditions experienced during walking. By considering both scenarios, the simulation is better equipped to reflect the complexities of human movement and the mechanical responses involved.

4.3 Results and Discussion

4.3.1 Mesh Convergence Results

The maximum von Mises stresses were systematically calculated for a range of applied pressure loads, specifically 0.1 MPa, 0.2 MPa, and 0.3 MPa. Throughout the analysis, a significant trend was observed in the induced stresses within the plantar region as the mesh density increased. Initially using a very coarse mesh consisting of 4,726 elements, the stress distribution exhibited notably high variability. This variability substantially decreased when transitioning to a fine mesh with 16,699 elements, where the stresses began to show a clearer pattern of convergence. This pattern was consistent across all specified pressure loads, highlighting a pronounced response of the stress distribution to the refinement of the mesh. As the mesh was further refined, from fine to very fine, comprising 21,916 elements, and subsequently to an even finer mesh with 27,834 elements, the maximum von Mises stresses began to stabilize. The values exhibited minimal variation under continued refinement,

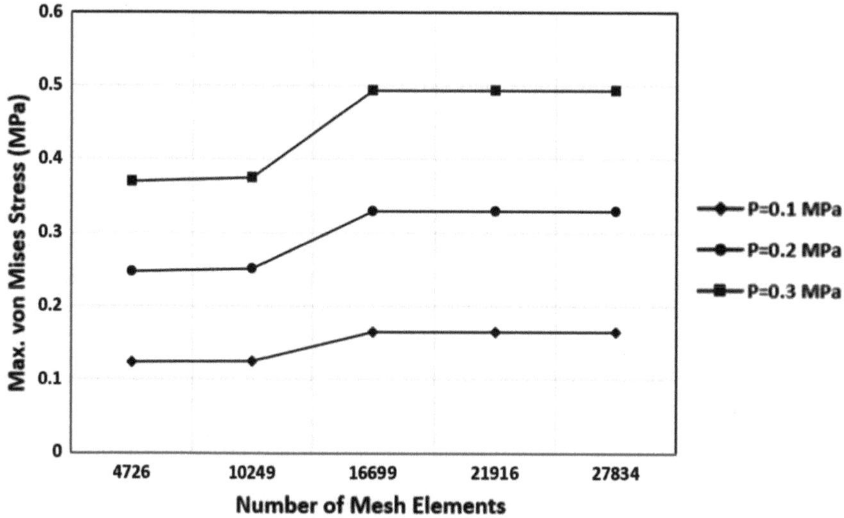

Fig. 4.4 Mesh convergence study results. *Reproduced with permission from IOP Science* [26]

suggesting that a threshold had been reached in terms of mesh density where additional elements yielded diminishing returns in accuracy of the stress readings. This behavior was visually supported by the data presented in Fig. 4.4, which illustrated the diminishing differences between the stress values across the various meshes under each loading condition. After conducting a thorough mesh convergence study, the fine mesh configuration, consisting of 16,699 elements, was determined to be the optimal choice for subsequent analyses. This selection ensured an effective balance between computational efficiency and the desired accuracy in the stress distribution evaluation, allowing for reliable results in further investigations of the material behavior under applied loads.

4.3.2 Plantar Stresses Due to Varying Ulcer Locations

A thorough analysis was conducted on all 52 ulcer sites, assessing each one individually to evaluate plantar stress distribution and calculate the maximum von Mises stress, as depicted in Fig. 4.5. This systematic approach allowed for a detailed understanding of how stress is distributed across various regions of the foot. The evaluation of the first four bands of ulcers, which are located on the forefoot at specific foot lengths of 0.1063, 0.1732, 0.2402, and 0.3071, revealed a stress distribution pattern that closely mimics that of a healthy, normal foot. Importantly, the analysis showed that maximum von Mises stress was concentrated at the periphery of the heel. This finding indicates a particular focal point of stress, which is likely to be a contributing factor in the development of ulcers in that area. In contrast, the first two ulcer locations identified on the big toe and the long toe showed notable deviations from this general stress distribution pattern. Specifically, these sites showed maximum stress values of +36% and −1.4%, respectively, when compared to the other ulcer locations. Such discrepancies suggest that the anatomical positions and specific loading patterns of these toes render them more vulnerable to stress-related injuries. The unique biomechanics of the forefoot, combined with the varying degrees of pressure applied during movement, could be instrumental in the heightened risk of ulcer formation in these areas. Overall, this analysis underscores the importance of understanding stress distribution in the foot, as it can provide valuable insights into preventing and managing ulcer development, particularly in vulnerable areas.

In the fifth band of ulcers, situated at the midfoot (specifically at 0.3740 of the foot length, with widths measuring 0.1460 and 0.3177), a pronounced increase in stress buildup was observed surrounding the ulcer sites. This was in addition to the already elevated stress levels at the periphery of the heel. These findings highlight the critical role of midfoot structural integrity in the development of ulcers, indicating that excessive pressure in this area can significantly worsen preexisting conditions and potentially lead to new ulcer formation. Furthermore, in the subsequent bands of ulcers located at foot lengths of 0.4409 and 0.5079, there was a dramatic escalation in stress accumulation around the ulcer sites, with stress values soaring by as much as 400% when compared to those associated with forefoot ulcers. Notably, while these stress levels increased, the stress at the heel remained relatively stable, suggesting that alterations in dynamic foot mechanics predominantly impact the forefoot and midfoot regions, rather than the heel. In the eighth band, which is positioned at 0.5748 of the foot length, with widths varying from 0.3177 to 0.8328, an astonishing 85% increase in maximum stress values was documented. This significant uptick in stress was accompanied by a substantial decrease of approximately 50% in stress at the heel corners. This finding indicates a possible redistribution of forces across the foot, which may be pivotal in shaping the risk factors associated with the emergence of new ulcers. Such alterations in stress distribution underscore the importance of careful monitoring and management of foot mechanics to mitigate the risk of ulcer development in vulnerable populations.

The ulcer identified in the tenth band of the hindfoot was measured at a length of 0.7087 and a width of 0.4894. This particular ulcer demonstrated a significant increase in maximum stress, rising by as much as 165% at its walls. In addition to this ulcer, several other heel ulcers were assessed at various lengths, 0.7756, 0.8425, 0.9094, and 0.9567, with corresponding widths of 0.2268, 0.3177, 0.3985, 0.4894, and 0.6611. These ulcers exhibited a significant rise in maximum von Mises stresses at their borders, with recorded values ranging from 0.72 MPa to 1.33 MPa. This variation in stress levels across different ulcer locations not only highlights the complexity of mechanical load distribution on the foot but also raises important concerns regarding the risk of tissue breakdown and the potential for new ulcer formation. Such insights are illustrated in Fig. 4.5, which visually represents these stress variations. The findings from this comprehensive analysis underscore the intricate dynamics of plantar stress and its crucial role in the development of foot ulcers.

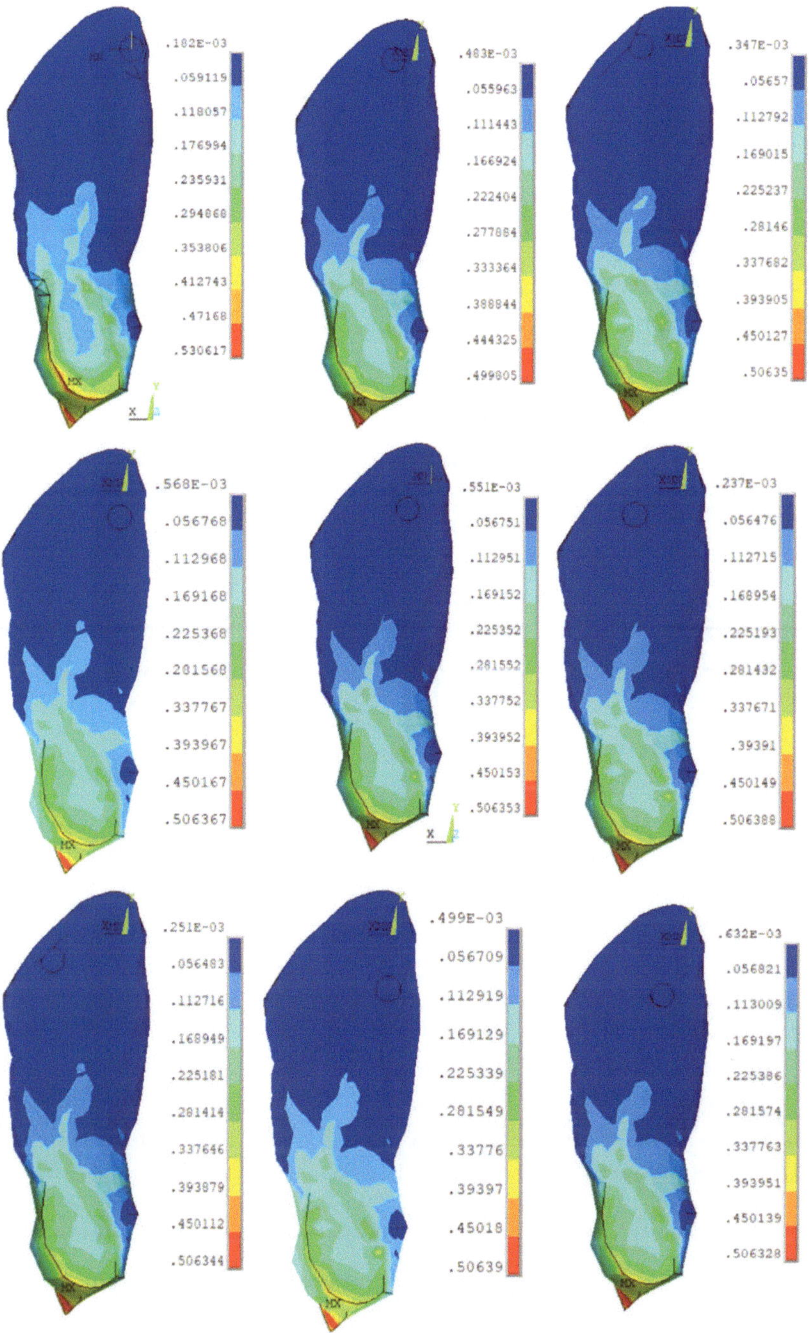

Fig. 4.5 Von Mises stress (MPa) simulation of foot ulcers at 52 different locations (starting from top-right in Fig. 4.2). *Reproduced with permission from IOP Science* [26]

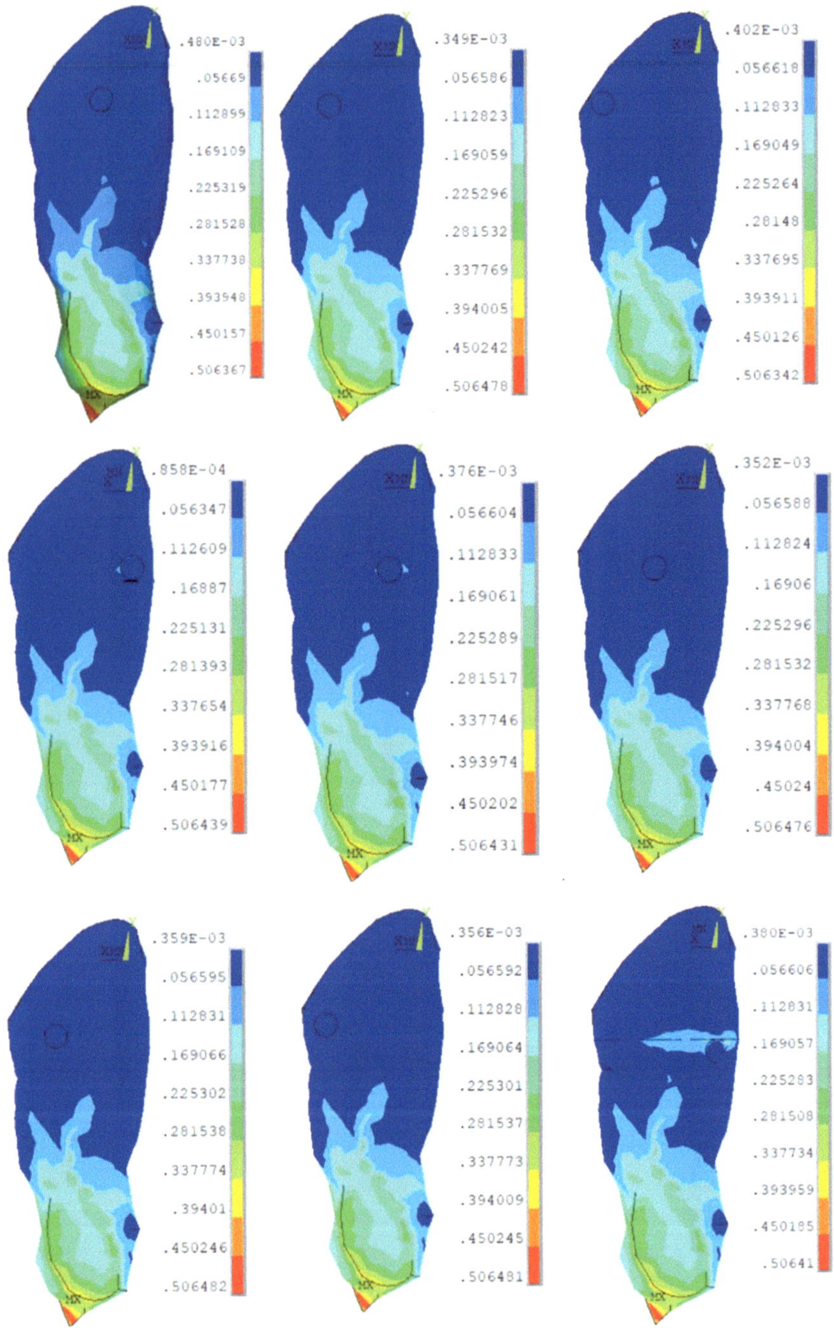

Fig. 4.5 (continued)

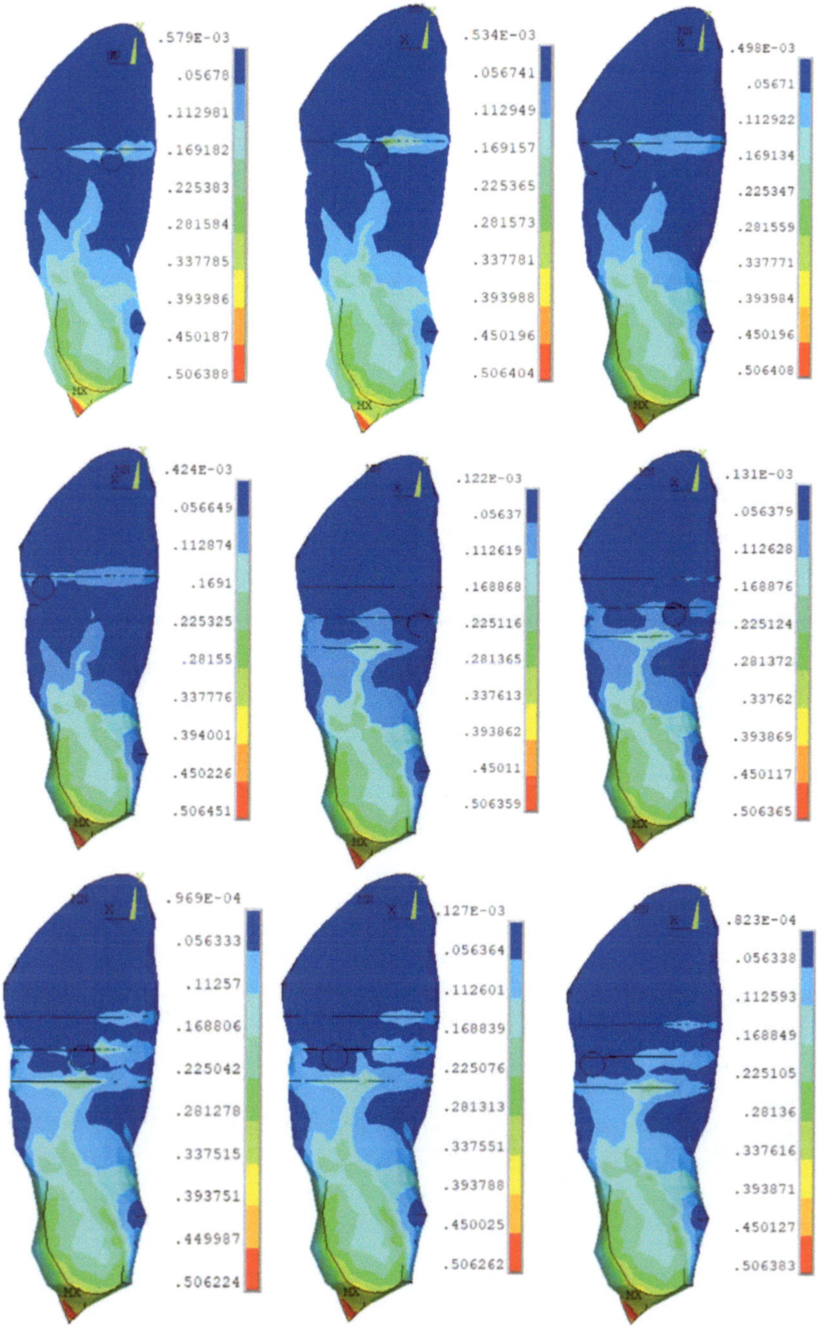

Fig. 4.5 (continued)

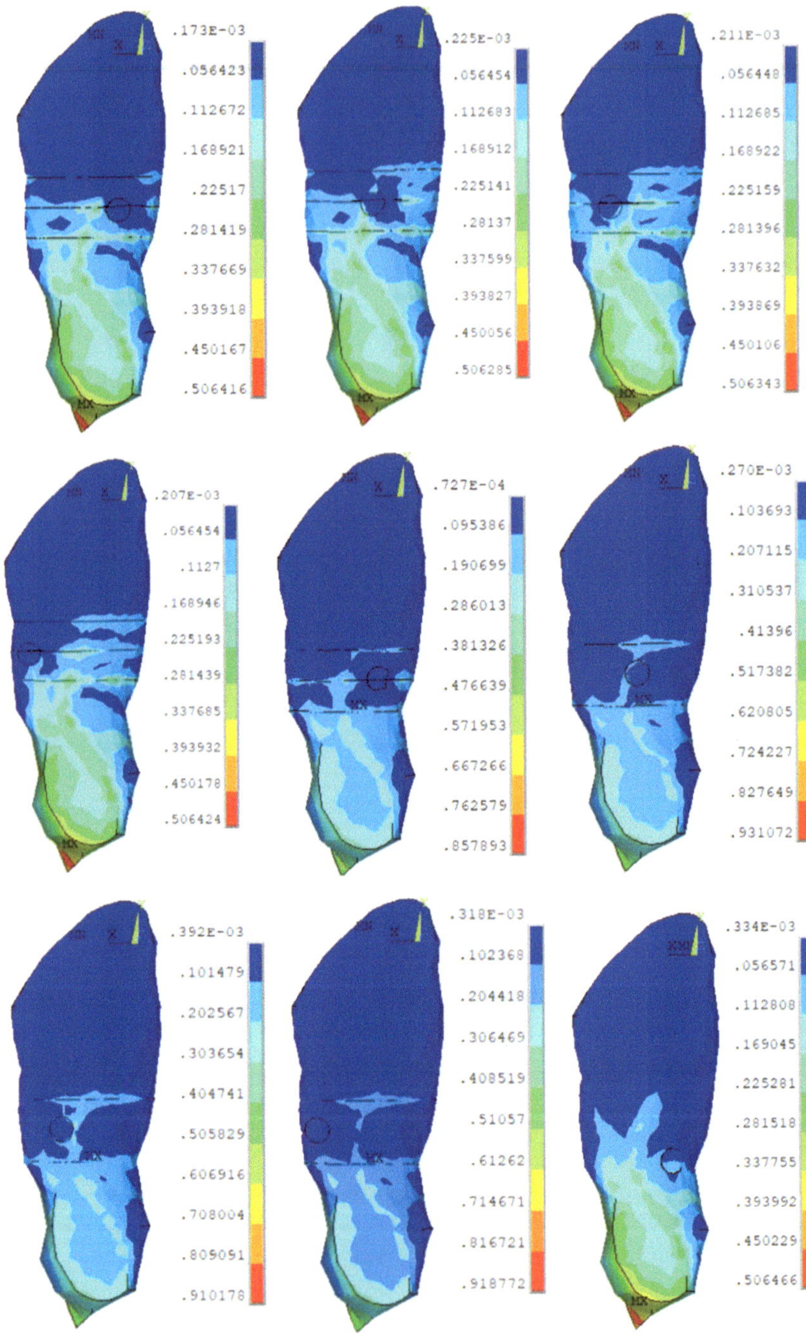

Fig. 4.5 (continued)

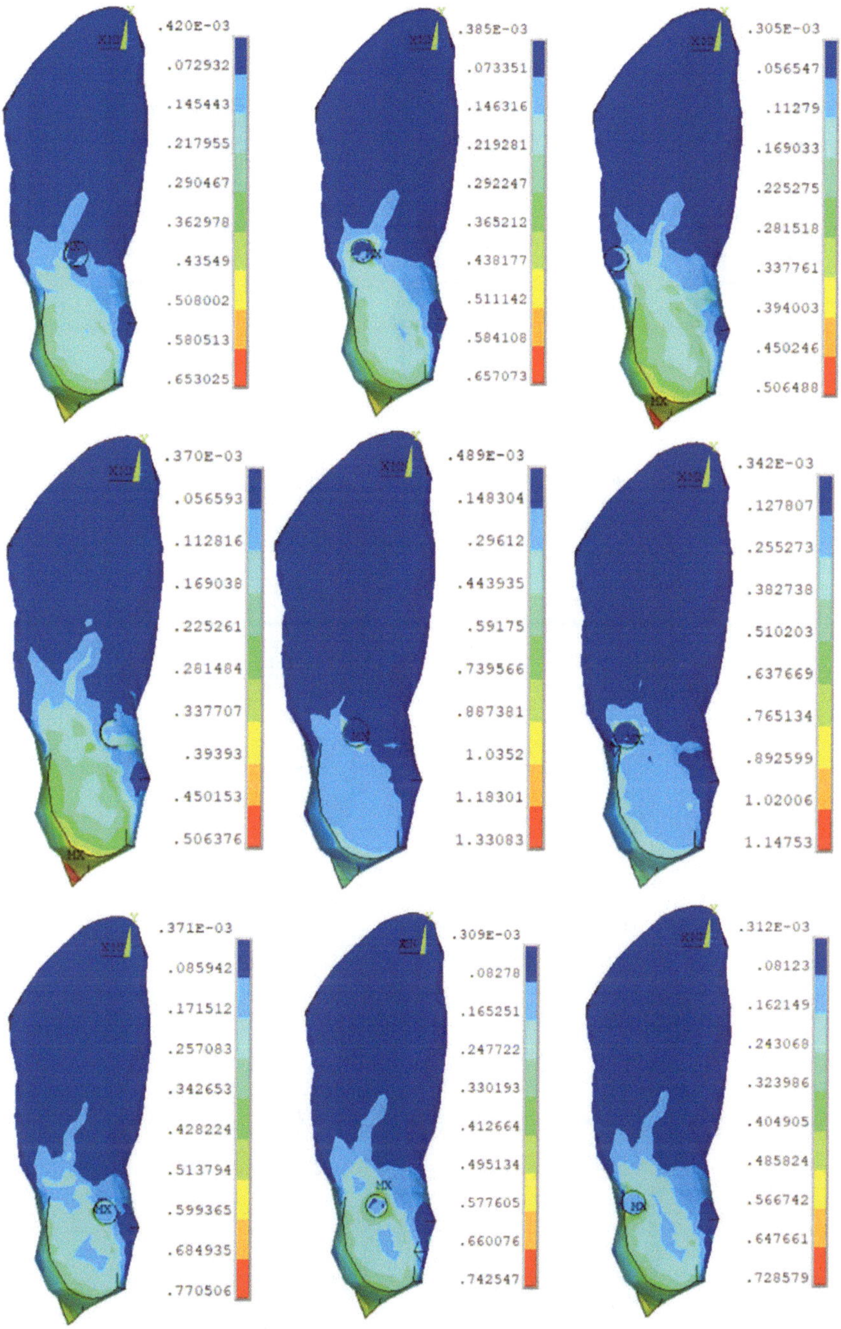

Fig. 4.5 (continued)

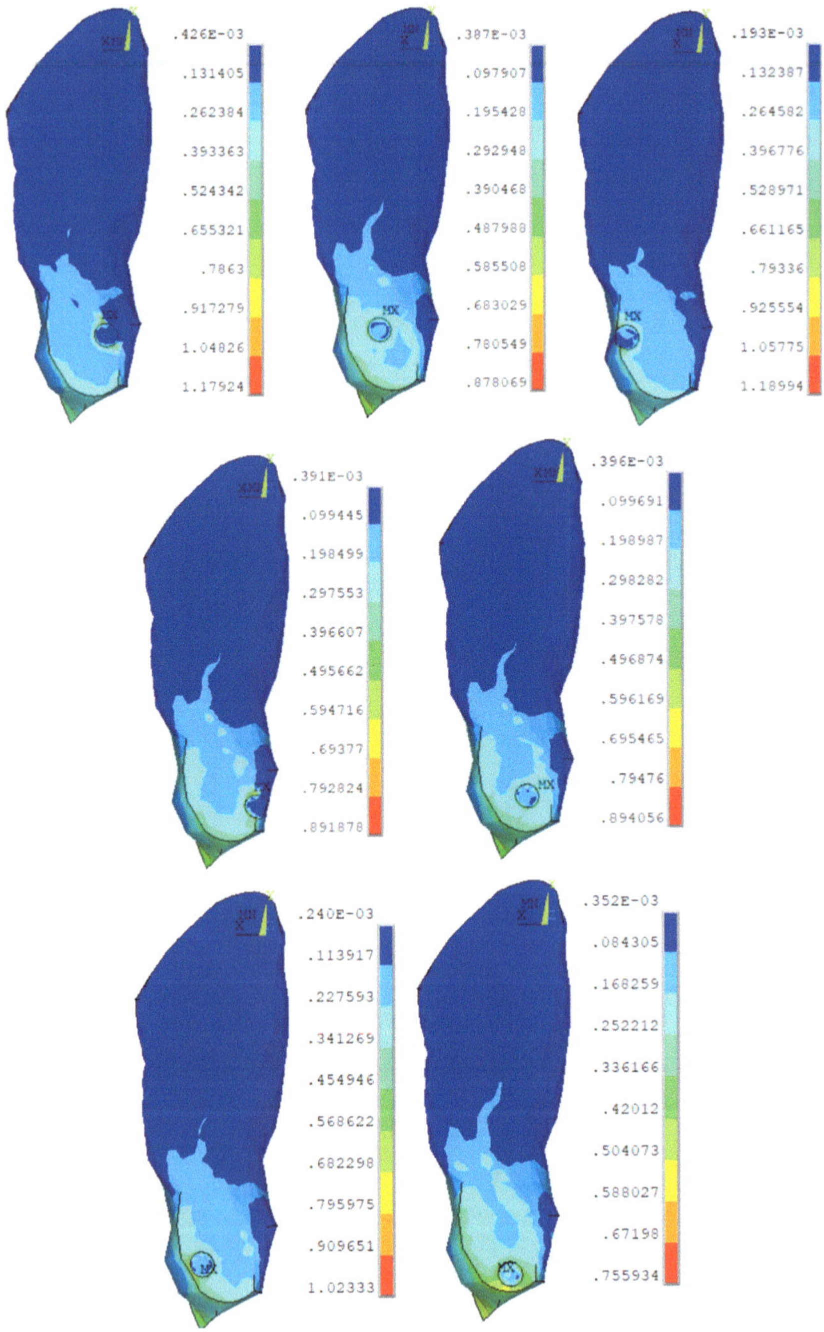

Fig. 4.5 (continued)

Understanding these patterns is vital for effective treatment and prevention strategies in individuals at risk of foot injuries and complications.

4.3.3 Local Ulcer Stresses Due to Varying Locations

The stresses observed at the walls of the ulcers were quantified at four specific locations: the top, bottom, left, and right sides. Our primary objective was to explore the potential for ulcer growth by closely analyzing these wall stress values. Notably, we found that ulcers initiating at a foot length of 0.2402 exhibited a marked upward trend in wall stresses. This suggests a shift in the dynamics of their development and raises concerns over their progression. For example, in the specific case of the ulcer located at a length of 0.2402 and a width of 0.1460, we discovered that the wall stress on the right side increased substantially, reaching levels nearly ten times greater than those observed on the other three sides. This increase in stress in that particular area indicates a heightened vulnerability and a concerning likelihood for continued ulcer growth. In addition, the group of ulcers situated in the midfoot area revealed consistently elevated stress values along their width. This raises alarm bells about the possibility of new ulcer sites forming in this critical region of the foot. Upon further investigation, it became evident that wall stresses for all midfoot ulcers were significantly heightened at one or two key locations around their perimeter. Such observations underscore the considerable risk of progressive ulcer growth, as these elevated stress values are likely to contribute to additional damage or promote the formation of new ulcers. These findings highlight the importance of closely monitoring these stress patterns, as they can provide critical insights into ulcer pathophysiology and guide preventive or therapeutic strategies to mitigate ulcer development and progression.

In the hindfoot region, our analysis revealed a substantial increase in maximum plantar stresses, with values soaring to as much as 20 times the normal levels. This dramatic elevation in stress corresponds with a notable rise in the stresses experienced by the ulcer walls. Across all four locations where we measured the ulcer walls, we recorded exceptionally high stress levels, which strongly indicates a heightened risk of ulcer progression in this vulnerable area. To provide a comprehensive overview of our findings, please consult Table 4.2. This table contains detailed measurements of ulcer wall stresses, along with projections on potential directions for growth, highlighting areas most susceptible to worsening. The data not only elucidates the mechanics behind ulcer formation but also emphasizes the critical importance of monitoring these stress levels to mitigate associated risks effectively. Understanding these factors is essential for developing targeted interventions to prevent ulcer progression and enhance patient outcomes.

Table 4.2 Ulcer wall stresses and possible growth direction. *Reproduced with permission from IOP Science* [26]

Ulcer location	Ulcer wall stress (MPa)				Possible growth direction
	Right	Top	Left	Bottom	
0.1460W, 0.1063L	0.0068	0.0020	0.0024	0.0070	Bottom
0.3177W, 0.1063L	0.0080	0.0022	0.0049	0.0046	Right
0.4894W, 0.1063L	0.0058	0.0030	0.0037	0.0058	Bottom
0.2015W, 0.1732L	0.0287	0.0078	0.0172	0.0091	Bottom
0.3177W, 0.1732L	0.0184	0.0075	0.0131	0.0111	Right
0.4894W, 0.1732L	0.0140	0.0043	0.0069	0.0131	Right
0.6611W, 0.1732L	0.0074	0.0020	0.0032	0.0055	Right
0.2015W, 0.2402L	0.0609	0.0010	0.0377	0.1140	Bottom
0.3177W, 0.2402L	0.0383	0.0875	0.0313	0.0304	Top
0.4894W, 0.2402L	0.0285	0.0116	0.0170	0.0251	Right
0.6611W, 0.2402L	0.0200	0.0076	0.0109	0.0080	Right
0.8328W, 0.2402L	0.0133	0.0057	0.0084	0.0102	Right
0.1460W, 0.3071L	0.0517	0.0907	0.0894	0.0278	Top
0.3177W, 0.3071L	0.1000	0.0083	0.0693	0.0010	Right
0.4894W, 0.3071L	0.0378	0.0135	0.0326	0.0118	Right
0.6611W, 0.3071L	0.0368	0.0143	0.0233	0.0235	Right
0.8328W, 0.3071L	0.0227	0.0143	0.0220	0.0200	Right
0.1460W, 0.3740L	0.1208	0.0749	0.1000	0.0060	Right, Left
0.3177W, 0.3740L	0.0820	0.0456	0.0823	0.0084	Left
0.4894W, 0.3740L	0.0720	0.1112	0.0533	0.0202	Top

(continued)

Table 4.2 (continued)

Ulcer location	Ulcer wall stress (MPa)				Possible growth direction
	Right	Top	Left	Bottom	
0.6611W, 0.3740L	0.0513	0.0057	0.0736	0.0544	Left, Right
0.8328W, 0.3740L	0.0553	0.0916	0.0378	0.0743	Top
0.1460W, 0.4409L	0.0075	0.0032	0.0095	0.0119	Bottom
0.3177W, 0.4409L	0.0179	0.0103	0.1053	0.0324	Left
0.4894W, 0.4409L	0.0174	0.0137	0.1013	0.1025	Bottom, Left
0.6611W, 0.4409L	0.0730	0.0093	0.0319	0.0300	Right
0.8328W, 0.4409L	0.0491	0.0300	0.0171	0.0645	Bottom
0.3177W, 0.5079L	0.0112	0.0248	0.0545	0.0201	Left
0.4894W, 0.5079L	0.0070	0.1330	0.4053	0.3222	Left, Bottom
0.6611W, 0.5079L	0.1683	0.0219	0.0519	0.1193	Right, Bottom
0.8328W, 0.5079L	0.0558	0.0390	0.0016	0.1100	Bottom
0.3177W, 0.5748L	0.0120	0.0229	0.0383	0.0253	Left, Bottom
0.4894W, 0.5748L	0.0138	0.1076	0.1180	0.1000	Left
0.6611W, 0.5748L	0.2424	0.2124	0.1200	0.2055	Right
0.8328W, 0.5748L	0.1020	0.1356	0.0712	0.0298	Top
0.3177W, 0.6417L	0.0254	0.0803	0.0812	0.1431	Bottom
0.4894W, 0.6417L	0.1326	0.1916	0.6530	0.2412	Left
0.6611W, 0.6417L	0.5667	0.2697	0.2178	0.4770	Right, Bottom
0.8328W, 0.6417L	0.1674	0.0281	0.0203	0.0310	Right

(continued)

Table 4.2 (continued)

Ulcer location	Ulcer wall stress (MPa)				Possible growth direction
	Right	Top	Left	Bottom	
0.3177W, 0.7087L	0.1105	0.1077	0.1256	0.2040	Left
0.4894W, 0.7087L	0.1509	0.02280	0.5555	1.3308	Bottom
0.6611W, 0.7087L	0.3462	0.2737	0.1665	1.1475	Bottom
0.3177W, 0.7756L	0.1631	0.0761	0.6617	0.3759	Left
0.4894W, 0.7756L	0.4327	0.7425	0.3988	0.5662	Top, Bottom
0.6611W, 0.7756L	0.4675	0.5769	0.0712	0.7285	Bottom
0.3177W, 0.8425L	0.1071	1.1792	0.3255	0.8752	Top, Bottom
0.4894W, 0.8425L	0.4592	0.7758	0.5704	0.3783	Top
0.6611W, 0.8425L	0.3687	1.189	0.0588	0.4958	Top, Bottom
0.2268W, 0.9094L	0.00283	0.8918	0.5816	0.7053	Top, Bottom
0.3985W, 0.909L	0.8940	0.3904	0.5055	0.3090	Right
0.5702W, 0.9094L	0.5515	0.4586	0.9477	1.0233	Bottom, Left
0.3985W, 0.9567L	0.3565	0.3408	0.7559	0.7027	Left, Bottom

4.3.4 Prediction of Maximum Plantar Stress and Its Location Due to Varying Ulcer Locations

A comprehensive analysis was performed utilizing a wide range of data points to develop a robust prediction model for ulcer formation on the foot. This study focused on the specific locations of ulcers, examining both the length and width of the foot, while also quantifying the maximum plantar stress experienced at these locations. Figure 4.6a and b illustrates the variation in mean maximum von Mises stress corresponding to the identified ulcer locations, providing a visual representation of the stress patterns. The findings revealed that ulcers located at the extreme ends of the foot's width, specifically the outer edges, tended to display the lowest mean maximum stress values. This observation suggests that these peripheral areas may be less prone to pressure-related damage, potentially due to their anatomical structure or the way weight is distributed during movement. However, for the ulcers positioned along the mid-section of the foot's width, the data did not show any consistent trends. This lack of a definitive pattern indicates a more intricate relationship between ulcer formation and pressure, warranting further detailed investigation to uncover the underlying factors contributing to these observations. In contrast, a significant trend emerged when examining the locations of ulcers along the length of the foot. Notably, ulcer sites originating from the midfoot exhibited progressively higher mean maximum stress values as they extended toward the hindfoot region. This trend culminated at the heel area, which consistently recorded the highest mean maximum stress levels across all measurements taken. This finding underscores the critical need to focus on pressure distribution when devising ulcer prevention strategies, particularly in the heel area, where the likelihood of ulceration appears to be considerably elevated. Overall, these insights emphasize the necessity for targeted interventions tailored to stress distribution patterns across both the length and width of the foot. Understanding these dynamics is essential for developing effective prevention and treatment strategies to mitigate the risk of ulcer formation, ultimately improving patient outcomes for individuals at risk.

The analysis of maximum stress locations on the foot was conducted by plotting data along both the width and length, as illustrated in Fig. 4.7a and b, respectively. The findings indicated that ulcers located on the lateral aspect of the foot exhibited a consistent pattern in their maximum stress locations. This suggests that, despite variations in individual cases, the stress distribution in this area remains relatively uniform, which could have implications for predicting ulcer formation and developing targeted interventions. Conversely, ulcers that appeared on the medial side of the foot showed marked variation in their maximum stress locations. This inconsistency implies that the mechanical forces acting on this region of the foot are more complex and may involve different factors compared to the lateral side. Understanding these nuanced differences is crucial for improving treatment strategies and preventive measures for foot ulcers, particularly in individuals with conditions that affect foot health, such as diabetes.

Upon closely examining ulcers situated along the length of the foot, it has become increasingly apparent that the areas experiencing the highest levels of stress are predominantly concentrated in the hindfoot, especially around the heel region. This observation indicates that the hindfoot is likely subjected to greater mechanical forces during daily activities such as walking, running, and standing. These heightened loads may play a significant role in the formation and exacerbation of ulcers in this vulnerable area. Moreover, understanding the specific distribution of these mechanical stresses is vital for the development of effective prevention strategies and treatment protocols for foot ulcers. By identifying the precise locations and conditions that lead to increased pressure, healthcare providers can implement more targeted interventions, such as customized footwear, specialized orthotics, and appropriate wound care measures, to mitigate the risk of ulcer development and promote overall foot health.

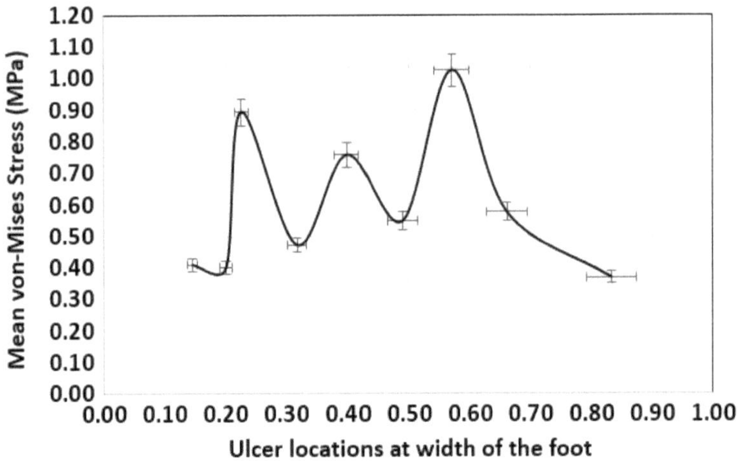

(a)

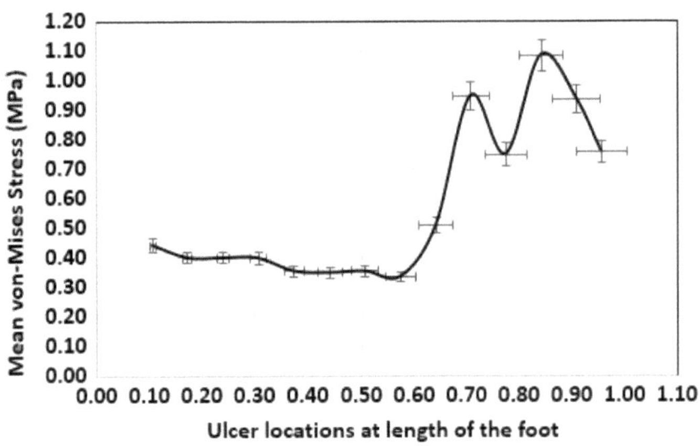

(b)

Fig. 4.6 Mean maximum von Mises stress (MPa) due to varying ulcer locations: **a** Along the width and **b** Along the length. *Reproduced with permission from IOP Science* [26]

Based on the detailed results and graphical representations shown in Figs. 4.6 and 4.7, we developed four specific equations aimed at determining the maximum plantar stress and identifying its precise location in relation to predefined ulcer coordinates. Equation 4.1 is designed to estimate the mean maximum von Mises stress that occurs across the width of the foot, specifically tailored to a given ulcer location defined by its position relative to foot width. By employing a three-term Fourier series for curve fitting, this equation achieved an impressive correlation coefficient of R2 = 0.968. This high value indicates a strong relationship between the model and actual data,

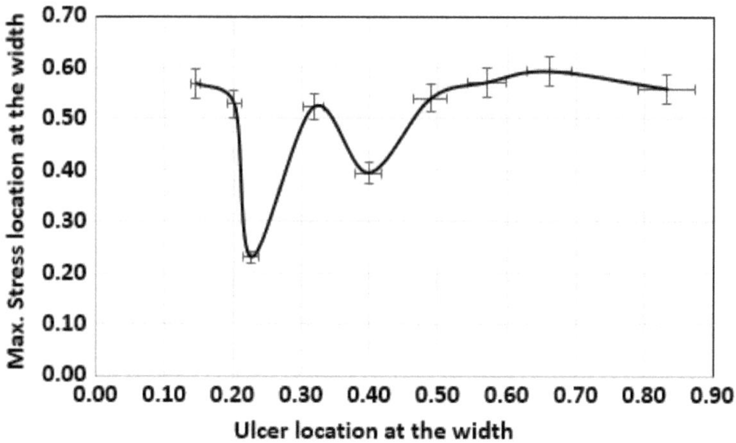

(a)

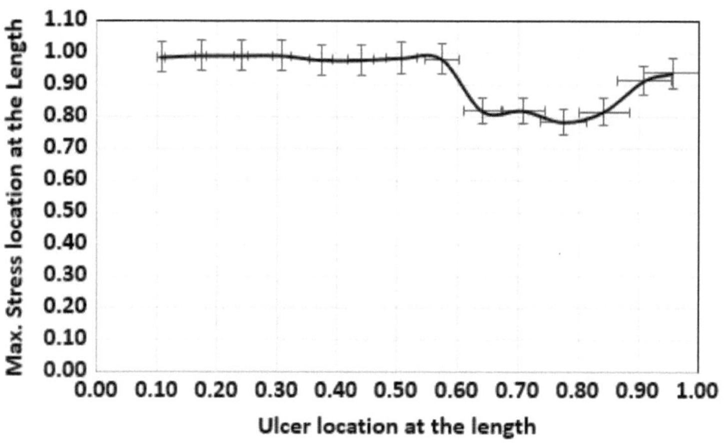

(b)

Fig. 4.7 Maximum von Mises stress (MPa) location due to varying ulcer locations: **a** Along the width and **b** Along the length. *Reproduced with permission from IOP Science* [26]

providing confidence that this equation can reliably predict stress levels based on the specified parameters of foot width. Such precision is crucial for understanding how stress distributions may contribute to the formation or exacerbation of ulcers in vulnerable patients. In a parallel manner, Eq. 4.2 quantifies the mean maximum von Mises stress along the length of the foot for ulcer locations defined concerning foot length. This equation utilizes a fifth-degree polynomial for curve fitting, yielding a correlation coefficient of R2 = 0.902. While this value is slightly lower than that of Eq. 4.1, it still reflects a good level of fit. This suggests that Eq. 4.2 is also a valuable tool, particularly when assessing the stress levels that occur longitudinally along the foot and could inform targeted interventions. The integration of these two equations offers a comprehensive framework for predicting plantar stress in relation to ulcer development. This predictive capability is essential for clinical assessments and can significantly enhance treatment planning in foot care. By understanding the factors contributing to maximum stress points, healthcare providers can devise more effective strategies to prevent ulcer formation and manage existing conditions, ultimately leading to improved patient outcomes.

$$\begin{aligned} \textit{Mean Max. Stress (Along Foot Width)} &= 0.6529 + 0.2701\cos(18.75x) \\ &+ (-1.607)\sin(18.75x) + (-0.073)\cos(37.5x) \\ &+ 0.2204\sin(37.5x) + (-0.0832)\cos(56.25x) + 0.3112\sin(56.25x) \end{aligned} \tag{4.1}$$

$$\begin{aligned} \textit{Mean Max. Stress (Along Foot Length)} &= -41.909\mathrm{x}^5 + 82.504\mathrm{x}^4 \\ &- 52.733\mathrm{x}^3 + 13.591\mathrm{x}^2 - 1.6234\,\mathrm{x} + 0.503 \end{aligned} \tag{4.2}$$

Equation 4.3 outlines a methodology for estimating the position of maximum stress along the width of the foot, using the known location of an ulcer as a reference point, which is expressed in terms of the foot's width. This predictive model was developed through a curve-fitting approach employing a three-term Gaussian function, which has demonstrated a robust correlation with empirical data, evidenced by an impressive R2 value of 0.985. Such a high degree of fit indicates that the model effectively captures the underlying relationship between the ulcer's location and the concomitant stress distribution across the foot's width, thereby offering valuable insights for clinicians in assessing potential areas of concern. In parallel, Eq. 4.4 is designed to estimate the location of maximum stress along the length of the foot, utilizing the ulcer position as a reference, expressed in terms of foot length. This model was fitted using a sixth-degree polynomial, resulting in an R2 value of 0.930. While this value also reflects a good fit, it is slightly lower than that of Eq. 4.3. This discrepancy suggests that there may be greater variability in the stress distribution along the foot's length compared to the width, which could have implications for how doctors approach treatment and prevention strategies. Together, these equations represent powerful analytical tools that facilitate the prediction of stress concentrations on the foot. Understanding these stress distributions is critical for ulcer management and prevention, as it allows healthcare providers to identify at-risk areas of the foot and implement targeted interventions to mitigate the risk of ulcer development. By refining our understanding of these relationships, we can improve patient outcomes and enhance the overall quality of care in managing foot health.

$$\begin{aligned} \textit{Mean Max. Stress Location (Along Foot Width)} &= 0.6118e^{\left(-\left(\frac{x-0.6871}{0.4603}\right)^2\right)} \\ &+ 1.389e^{\left(-\left(\frac{x-0.1725}{0.02413}\right)^2\right)} \\ &+ 0.257e^{\left(-\left(\frac{x-0.3034}{0.02909}\right)^2\right)} \end{aligned} \tag{4.3}$$

$$\text{Mean Max. Stress Location (Along Foot Length)} = -132.71x^6 + 415.23x^5 - 497.11x^4 + 287.14x^3 - 83.527x^2 + 11.439x + 0.4219 \quad (4.4)$$

4.4 Conclusions

In conclusion, the study's findings revealed that ulcers situated on the forefoot were closely associated with significant stress concentrations at the corners of the heel. This correlation highlights a potential risk for the development of new ulcers in these high-stress areas, drawing attention to the complex and interconnected nature of foot anatomy and the mechanisms behind ulcer formation. Notably, while the different locations of forefoot ulcers did not produce distinct variations in the maximum stresses generated or their specific locations, clear differences emerged when examining midfoot and hindfoot ulcers. Ulcers located in the midfoot region demonstrated comparatively low stress concentrations, suggesting that these areas may carry a reduced risk of complications such as further ulceration. Conversely, hindfoot ulcers showed high stress concentrations at their walls, which indicates an increased likelihood of ulcer growth and deterioration due to the elevated forces acting on these areas. These findings are consistent with earlier literature, underscoring the significance of understanding the biomechanical factors that contribute to DFUs [22]. Such insights are essential for identifying at-risk areas of the foot, which can inform clinical decisions. Furthermore, the data obtained from these simulations underwent rigorous analysis to establish precise relationships between peak stress values, the locations where these peaks occurred, and the specific ulcer sites. This comprehensive understanding is vital for designing targeted interventions and developing preventive strategies aimed at managing and reducing the risk of further ulcerations in diabetic patients, ultimately improving their overall foot health and quality of life.

References

1. Aumiller WD, Dollahite HA (2015) Pathogenesis and management of diabetic foot ulcers. J Am Acad Physician Assist. 28:28–34
2. Boulton AJM (2008) The diabetic foot: grand overview, epidemiology and pathogenesis. Diabetes Metab Res Rev 24:S3–S6
3. Prompers L et al. Resource utilisation and costs associated with the treatment of diabetic foot ulcers. Prospective data from the Eurodiale Study. Diabetologia 51, 1826–1834
4. Ibrahim M, El Hilaly R, Taher M, Morsy A (2013) A pilot study to assess the effectiveness of orthotic insoles on the reduction of plantar soft tissue strain. Clin Biomech 28:68–72
5. Lazzarini PA et al (2015) Prevalence of foot disease and risk factors in general inpatient populations: A systematic review and meta-analysis. BMJ Open 5:e008544

6. Monteiro-Soares M et al (2020) Diabetic foot ulcer classifications: A critical review. Diabetes Metab Res Rev 36:e3272
7. Prompers L et al (2007) High prevalence of ischaemia, infection and serious comorbidity in patients with diabetic foot disease in Europe. Baseline results from the Eurodiale study. Diabetologia 50, 18–25
8. Owings TM et al (2009) Plantar pressures in diabetic patients with foot ulcers which have remained healed. Diabet Med 26:1141–1146
9. Veves A, Murray HJ, Young MJ, Boulton AJM (1992) The risk of foot ulceration in diabetic patients with high foot pressure: a prospective study. Diabetologia 35:660–663
10. Singh G, Chanda A (2024) Finite element modeling of diabetic foot: a state-of-the-art review. Eng Res Express 6:012507
11. Kogani M, Mansournia MA, Doosti-Irani A, Holakouie-Naieni K (2015) Risk factors for amputation in patients with diabetic foot ulcer in southwest Iran: a matched case-control study. Epidemiol. Health 37:e2015044
12. Jeong E-G et al (2018) Depth and combined infection is important predictor of lower extremity amputations in hospitalized diabetic foot ulcer patients. Korean J Intern Med 33:952–960
13. Bus SA et al (2016) IWGDF guidance on footwear and offloading interventions to prevent and heal foot ulcers in patients with diabetes. Diabetes Metab Res Rev 32:25–36
14. Fernando ME et al (2016) Plantar pressures are higher in cases with diabetic foot ulcers compared to controls despite a longer stance phase duration. BMC Endocr Disord 16:51
15. Kaufman J, Breeding L, Rosenberg N (1987) Anatomic location of acute diabetic foot infection: Its influence on the outcome of treatment. Am Surg 53:109–112
16. Lavery LA, Armstrong DG, Harkless LB (1996) Classification of diabetic foot wounds. J Foot Ankle Surg 35:528–531
17. Cheung JTM, Zhang M, Leung AKL, Fan YB (2005) Three-dimensional finite element analysis of the foot during standing—a material sensitivity study. J Biomech 38:1045–1054
18. Telfer S, Erdemir A, Woodburn J, Cavanagh PR (2014) What has finite element analysis taught us about diabetic foot disease and its management? A Systematic Review. PLoS One 9:e109994
19. Zhang P et al (2017) Global epidemiology of diabetic foot ulceration: a systematic review and meta-analysis†. Annals of Medicine. 49 106–116 at https://doi.org/10.1080/07853890.2016.1231932
20. Marzoq A, Shiaa N, Zaboon R, Baghlany Q, Alabbood MH (2019) Assessment of the outcome of diabetic foot ulcers in basrah, southern Iraq: a cohort study. Int J Diabetes Metab. 25:33–38
21. Singh G, Gupta S, Chanda A (2021) Biomechanical modelling of diabetic foot ulcers: A computational study. J Biomech 127:110699
22. Chanda A, Unnikrishnan V (2018) Novel insole design for diabetic foot ulcer management. Proc Inst Mech Eng Part H J Eng Med 232, 1182–1195
23. Singh G, Lamba A, Chanda A (2024) Role of additive manufacturing for the management of diabetic foot ulcers. In Addit Manuf Biomed Appl 19–38 (Springer, Singapore). https://doi.org/10.1007/978-981-97-5456-4_2
24. Gupta S et al (2023) Diabot: development of a diabetic foot pressure tracking device. J 6, 32–47
25. Chhikara K, Singh G, Gupta S, Chanda A (2022) Progress of additive manufacturing in fabrication of foot orthoses for diabetic patients: A review. Ann 3D Print Med 8, 100085
26. Gupta S, Singh G, Chanda A (2021) Prediction of diabetic foot ulcer progression: a computational study. Biomed Phys Eng Express 7:065020
27. Bose D, Singh G, Gupta S, Chanda A (2024) Development of a novel customized insole for effective pressure offloading in diabetic patients. Prosthesis 6:341–356
28. Singh G, Bose D, Chanda A (2025) Development and testing of a novel diabetic orthosis for plantar pressure reduction. Facta Univ Ser Mech Eng. https://doi.org/10.22190/FUME240725044S
29. Besse JL, Leemrijse T, Deleu PA (2011) Diabetic foot: The orthopedic surgery angle. Orthopaedics and Traumatology: Surgery and Research. 97 314–329 at https://doi.org/10.1016/j.otsr.2011.03.001

30. Frykberg RG (2002) Diabetic foot ulcers: pathogenesis and management. American Family Physician 66
31. Singh G, Chanda A (2022) Biomechanical modeling of progressive wound healing: A computational study. Biomed Eng Adv. 4:100055
32. Chanda A, Upchurch W (2018) Biomechanical modeling of wounded skin. J Compos Sci 2, Page 69 2, 69
33. Gupta V, Singh G, Chanda A (2023) Modeling of metamaterial based incision patterns for generating high expansions in skin grafts. Clin Biomech 110:106118
34. Cheung JT-M, Zhang M (2008) Parametric design of pressure-relieving foot orthosis using statistics-based finite element method. Med Eng Phys 30:269–277
35. Chen W-M, Lee T, Lee PV-S, Lee JW, Lee S-J (2010) Effects of internal stress concentrations in plantar soft-tissue—A preliminary three-dimensional finite element analysis. Med Eng Phys 32:324–331

Chapter 5
Biomechanical Modeling of Progressive Wound Healing

Skin injuries are among the most prevalent types of injuries, often manifesting as wounds or cuts. The process of wound healing is intricate, involving a series of mechanical and biochemical mechanisms that begin with the formation of a clot at the injury site. While extensive research has been conducted on the micro-level cellular processes involved in wound healing, investigations into the macro-level biomechanics have primarily focused on standardized wound shapes and sizes, leaving a gap in our understanding of more complex wound geometries [1–3]. In this chapter, we introduced an approach by employing the finite element modeling (FEM) method to model realistic wound geometries for the first time. This advanced modeling allows us to analyze and characterize the stresses and strains that arise from the skin's inherent tension during the various phases of wound healing. We studied a diverse range of wound types, including diabetic wounds, venous ulcers, pressure sores, and other complex ulcerations, providing a comprehensive view of the healing process. By comparing the induced stresses across different healing phases for each wound type, we have gained valuable insights into the dynamic nature of wound healing. This knowledge is essential for pre-surgical planning and the implementation of robotic surgeries, as it informs the selection of appropriate wound closure techniques. Such techniques are crucial to ensure that the skin tissue is not overstressed, which can lead to complications like tearing or delayed healing. We anticipate that the findings from this work will pave the way for significant advancements in wound healing research. By delivering novel insights into the mechanics of wound healing, we aim to enhance the overall effectiveness of treatment strategies, ultimately improving patient outcomes and promoting faster recovery times.

A. Chanda and G. Singh, *Diabetic Foot Ulcer*, Biomedical Materials for Multi-functional Applications, https://doi.org/10.1007/978-981-95-2484-6_5

5.1 Introduction

Human skin possesses intricate mechanical properties that are essential for its function and resilience; it is characterized as nonlinear, anisotropic, viscoelastic, and incompressible. These properties are important for the skin to adapt to various stresses and strains encountered during daily activities [4, 5]. The skin is composed of three primary layers: the epidermis, which serves as the outer protective barrier; the dermis, which houses blood vessels, nerves, and connective tissue; and the hypodermis, which comprises fatty tissue that provides insulation and cushioning. The total thickness of skin can vary significantly, ranging from 1 to 4 mm depending on the specific body region [6, 7]. Wounds in the skin represent a major health issue, impacting a significant portion of the population at some point in their lives. These wounds can result from a wide array of factors, including poor blood circulation, which compromises healing; physical injuries such as cuts or abrasions; infections that can complicate recovery; tumors that may necessitate surgical removal; and surgical incisions themselves, which can sometimes lead to delayed healing. To improve understanding and treatment, wounds can be classified in several ways: by their type, such as diabetic ulcers, venous ulcers, and pressure ulcers, which relate to their origin; by underlying medical conditions, differentiating between ischemic (caused by inadequate blood supply) and nonischemic conditions, or between infected and non-infected wounds; and by healing duration, making a distinction between acute wounds (which heal in a timely manner) and chronic wounds (which persist over an extended period) [8, 9]. Wound healing involves a series of complex biological processes that operate at multiple scales, from micro-level cellular repairs to macro-level tissue regeneration. Understanding the biochemical and biomechanical mechanisms underlying these processes is critical for developing effective treatment strategies. This includes insights into the inflammatory response, tissue remodeling, and the role of growth factors, which together inform clinicians on how to best promote healing and restore skin integrity.

Biochemical wound healing is an intricate physiological process in which the dermis, the essential load-bearing layer of the skin, is meticulously rebuilt following an injury. This rebuilding is primarily facilitated by fibroblasts, which play a critical role in collagen deposition and tissue contraction [10]. The healing process begins with the formation of cytokine gradients that are activated during the initial inflammatory response [11]. Wound healing can be divided into four distinct but interrelated stages: hemostasis, inflammation, proliferation (characterized by new tissue formation), and maturation, which involves tissue remodeling [12] (Fig. 5.1). In the hemostasis phase, the body swiftly responds to the injury by forming a fibrin-rich clot composed mainly of platelets. This clot not only serves to prevent excessive blood loss but also provides a provisional scaffold that promotes cell migration toward the wound site. Following hemostasis, the inflammation stage occurs, typically within minutes to a few days post-injury. During this critical phase, various cellular species, including inflammatory cells such as neutrophils and macrophages, are attracted to the wound. Their primary roles involve clearing pathogens and debris, as well as facilitating the formation of the blood clot through the release of growth factors that stimulate cellular activity [13, 14]. The proliferation phase, which lasts from a few days to several weeks, is characterized by the active secretion of collagen by fibroblasts. This marks the creation of a new extracellular matrix (ECM), which gradually replaces the temporary fibrin clot. As the proliferative phase progresses, the epidermis begins to re-epithelialize, and the collagen ECM takes over from the fibrin clot, thereby supporting further tissue repair [15, 16]. Lastly, the remodeling phase, which can extend over months to years, focuses on re-establishing the collagen network. During this phase, the collagen fibers undergo restructuring and realignment, allowing the skin to restore its tensile strength and return to its natural state. This gradual remodeling is crucial for ensuring that the healing scar matures properly and that the skin regains its functionality and appearance [17, 18].

At a macro level, the study of wound healing biomechanics holds significant promise for improving surgical practices and establishing more effective guidelines for robotic suturing techniques. Given the ethical and biosafety concerns associated with conducting experiments on human skin, finite element (FE) analysis has emerged as a crucial tool for investigating the complex processes involved in wound closure [20–23]. The pioneering work in this area began in 1986 with Larrabee et al. [24], who developed the first two-dimensional FE model specifically designed to analyze wound closure mechanics. Their model established a FE matrix that

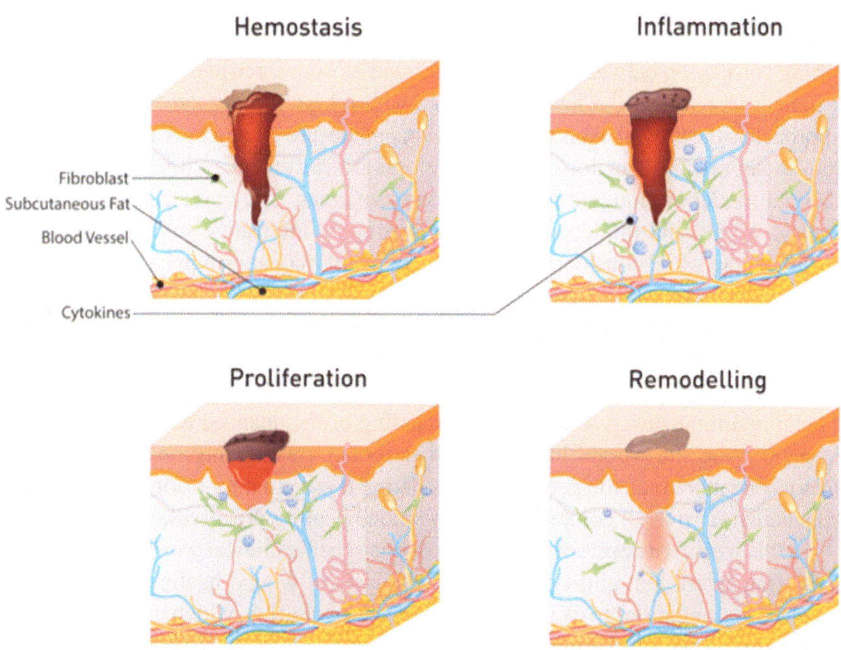

Fig. 5.1 Stages of wound healing of the skin. *Reproduced under the terms of the Creative Commons Attribution 4.0 International License* [19]

accurately captures the intricate deformation of skin during the healing process. This foundational work paved the way for subsequent studies, including those by Cavicchi et al. [25], who advanced the FE modeling approach by incorporating the effects of pre-stress. Pre-stress arises from the skin's natural tension, which has been shown to significantly influence both skin wrinkling and the overall dynamics of wound closure. Cavicchi et al. modeled the skin as a two-dimensional surface with isotropic material properties, applying biaxial pre-stress loads to two distinct circular wound sizes, i.e., large and small. Their findings indicated that the maximum stress experienced around the large wound was approximately 200 kPa higher than that surrounding the smaller wound, clearly demonstrating that the size of the wound plays a critical role in influencing the mechanical stresses imparted on the surrounding tissues.

Following this, Flynn et al. [11] expanded the understanding of wound mechanics by developing an FE model to assess the impact of different surgical excision shapes on wound closure dynamics. They examined four specific excision shapes: elliptical, circular, fusiform, and lazy S-plasty, under conditions of biaxial skin pre-stress set at 10 kPa along the X-axis (the long edge of the wound) and 5 kPa along the Y-axis (the short edge). Their analysis revealed that the elliptical excision required the least force for effective wound closure, suggesting that the geometric shape of a wound can significantly influence closure efficiency and healing outcomes. In 2012, Capek et al. [26] further refined the investigation by exploring the relationship between wound closure force and varying sizes of elliptical wounds, assessing conditions both with and without the influence of skin pre-stress. Their research indicated a strong correlation between the required wound closure force and both the size of the elliptical wound and the level of skin pre-stress, highlighting the need for tailored approaches in surgical excision and subsequent closure strategies. Chanda et al. [27] took a significant leap forward by developing a novel three-dimensional computational model to simulate multilayer skin dynamics. They created a symmetrical dermal wound and implemented suturing using an innovative suture pulling technique, all the while considering the implications of biaxial skin pre-stress. By simulating various suturing steps, they were able to predict the forces at play across the different stages of wound closure through complex numerical formulations. Despite these advancements, it is important to note that existing computational models of wound closure have predominantly utilized simplified, idealized wound geometries. This limitation restricts a deeper understanding of the nuanced mechanics involved in patient-specific wound healing. Further research expanding on patient-specific factors and more realistic geometrical modeling is essential for bridging this gap and enhancing our overall comprehension of wound healing processes.

In this work, we developed realistic, patient-specific clinical wound models using a FE framework that allows for detailed analysis of wound healing dynamics. We conducted simulations to examine various stages of clotting, which include the initial hemostatic response, clot maturation, and eventual resolution. Additionally, we characterized the effects of the skin's biaxial natural tension, which plays a critical role in how the tissue responds to injury and affects the healing process. Our in-depth analysis focused on the stresses generated in both the skin and the clot during the healing process. By varying the wound geometries, we aimed to understand how these differences influence healing effectiveness at different stages. The results of this study provide vital insights that can predict the condition of a clot depending on a specific healing stage and the unique geometry of the wound. Ultimately, this information is expected to serve as a valuable resource for healthcare professionals, particularly doctors and surgeons. By offering an objective assessment of wound healing effectiveness tailored to individual patient characteristics, practitioners will be better equipped to administer suitable and effective treatments. This research holds promise for improving clinical outcomes in wound care management by integrating biomechanical insights into the decision-making process.

5.2 Materials and Methods

5.2.1 Geometrical Modeling

The geometry of the wounds was carefully plotted on an XY graph, where precise coordinates were designated for the modeling of three-dimensional (3D) skin-wound models using Ansys APDL 2019 R2, a software developed in Canonsburg, Pennsylvania, USA. The process of developing the geometrical model for the skin wound comprised two distinct yet interconnected steps. In the first step, the two primary layers of the skin, the epidermis and the dermis, were modeled. The epidermis, the outermost layer, was set to a thickness of 0.1 mm, while the dermis, located beneath it, was assigned a thickness of 1.9 mm, resulting in a total skin model thickness of 2 mm. These measurements were carefully selected based on extensive literature to ensure biological accuracy and relevance [5, 23, 28]. In the subsequent step, various wound geometries were created on this two-layer skin model. Using the traced coordinates from the initial graph, the areas designated for the wounds were plotted directly onto the surface of the epidermal layer. To define the boundaries of these areas, the coordinates were connected using splines, creating a clear outline of the wound. Once the wound area was established, the next phase involved extruding this area to generate a 3D volume. This volume was created to a depth of 1 mm, effectively extending down to the midpoint of the two-layer skin model. A Boolean operation was then employed to subtract this volume from the skin model, forming a wound with a depth of exactly 1 mm. Table 5.1 provides a compilation of realistic images depicting the various wound types, the corresponding traced coordinates, and the resulting two-layer skin models. It is important to note that the area of the skin model was strategically selected to accommodate each wound geometry in a central position, allowing for accurate representation and analysis. The study focused on several categories of wounds, specifically diabetic wounds, venous ulcers, pressure sores, and other types of ulcerative wounds, providing comprehensive insights into their geometric characteristics and implications for healing.

Table 5.1 Wounds with traced geometrical coordinates and 3D wounded skin models. *Reproduced under the terms of the Creative Commons Attribution 4.0 International License* [19]

Realistic Wound	Wound Trace (Coordinates)	Geometrical Model
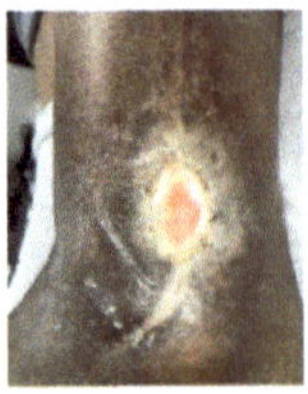	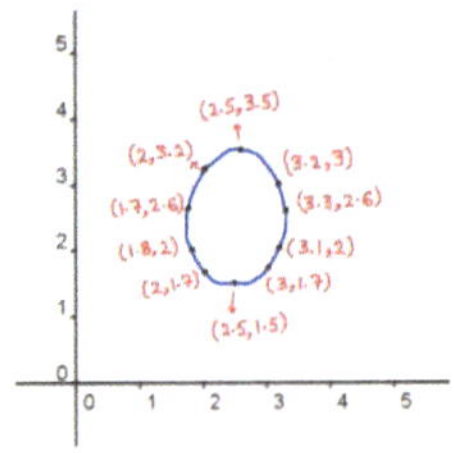	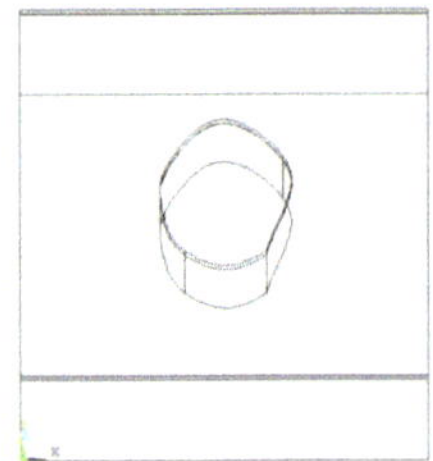
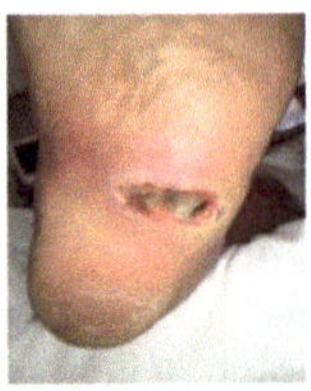	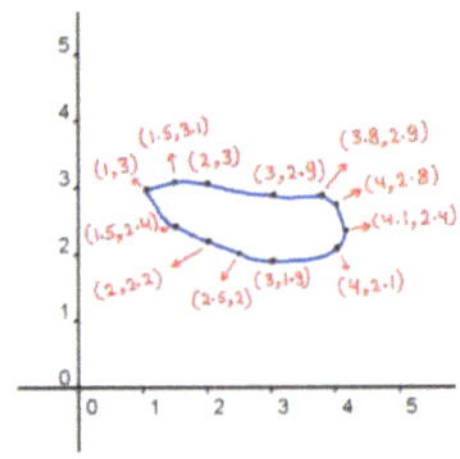	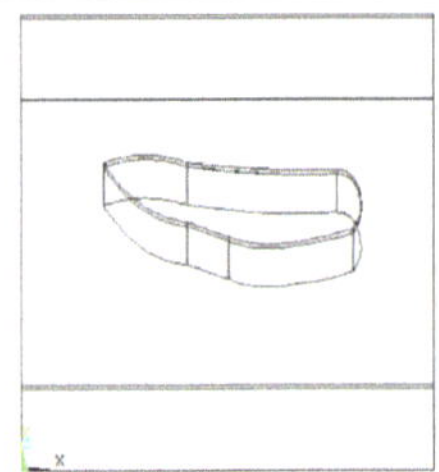
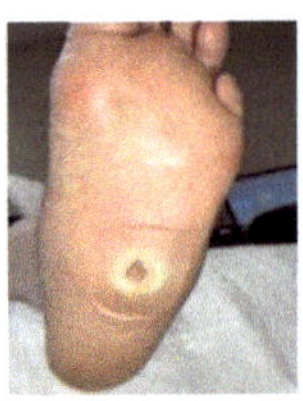	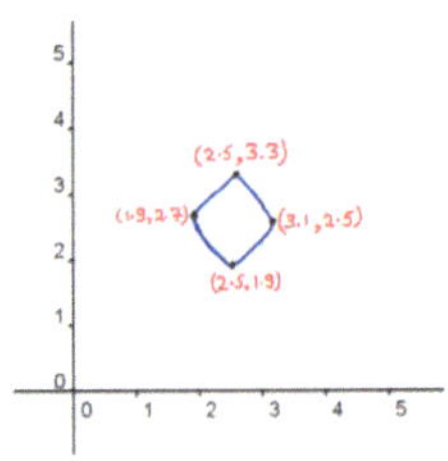	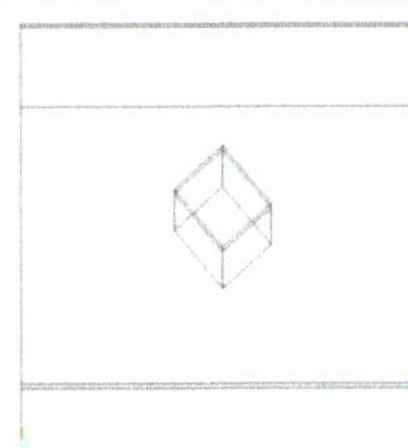
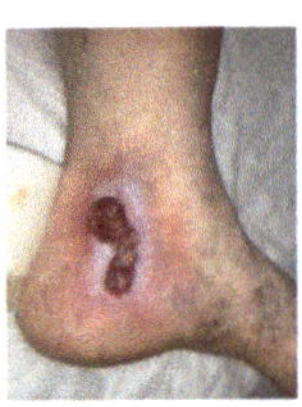	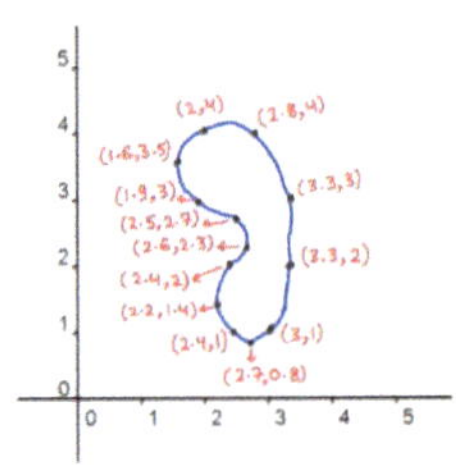	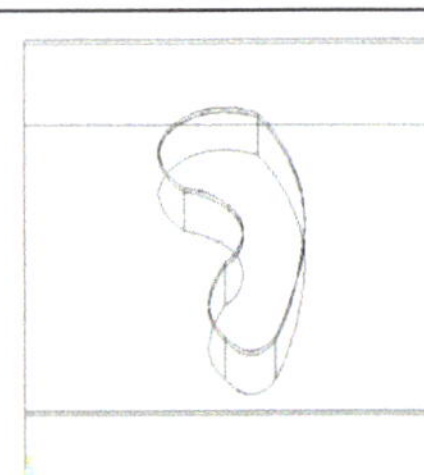
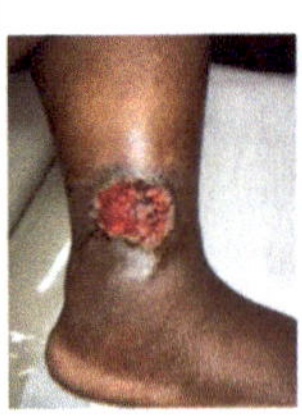	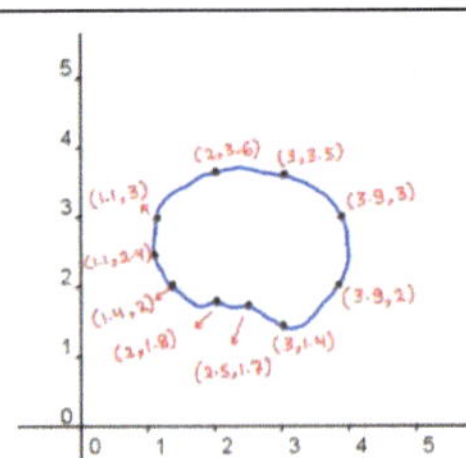	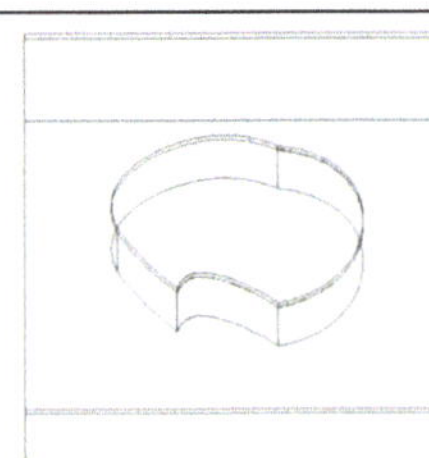

(continued)

Table 5.1 (continued)

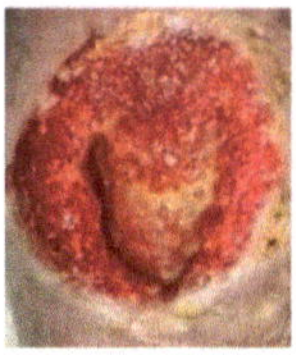	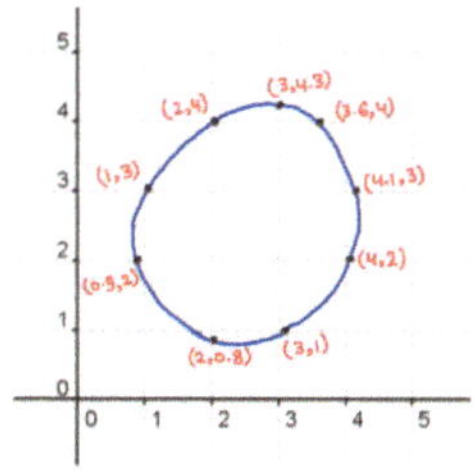	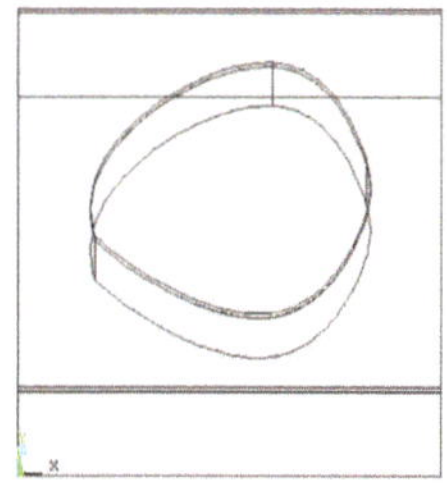
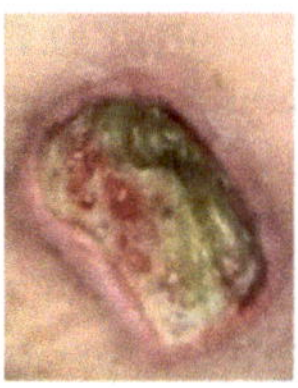	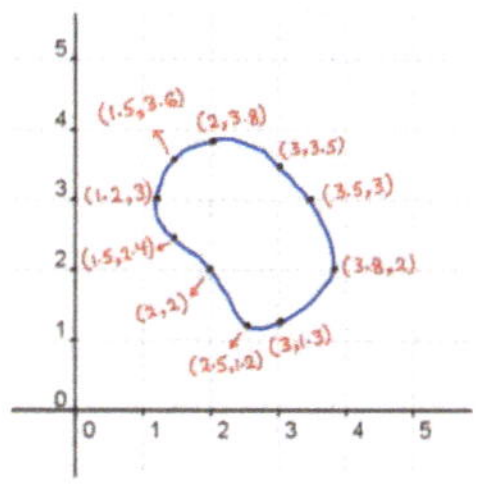	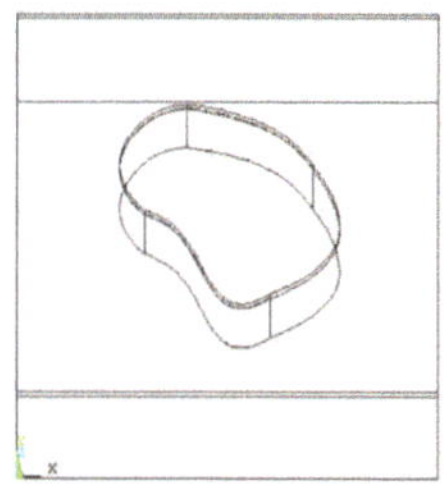
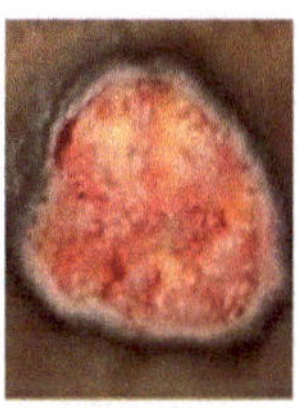	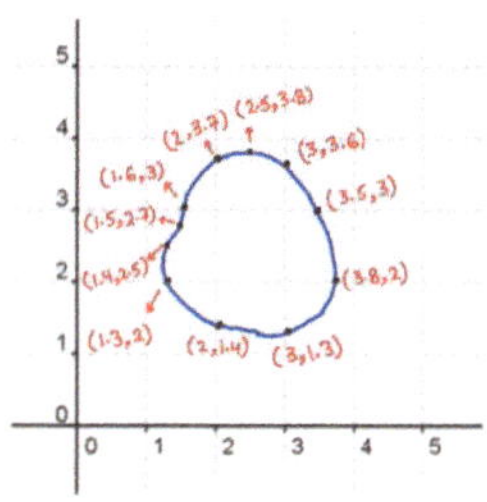	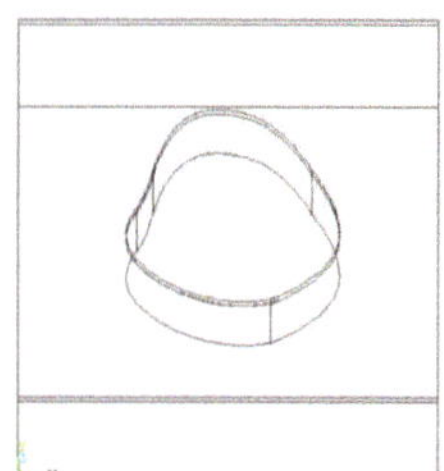
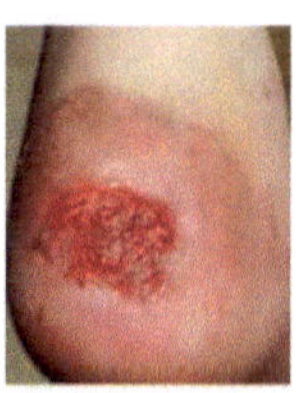	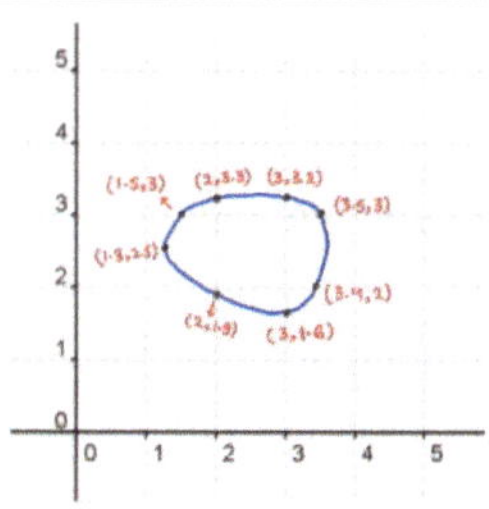	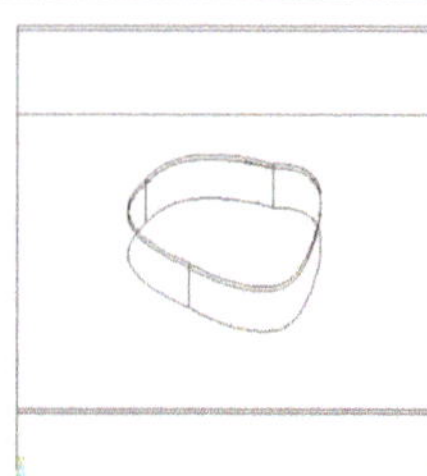
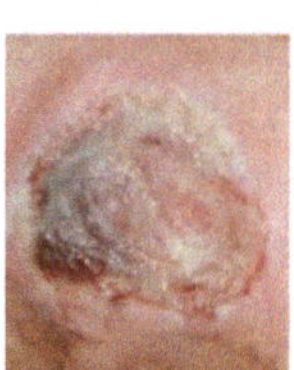	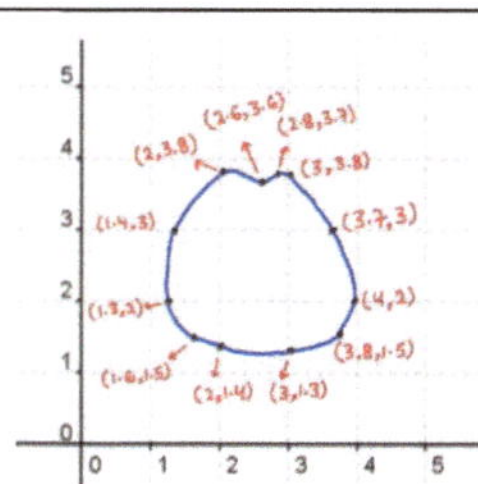	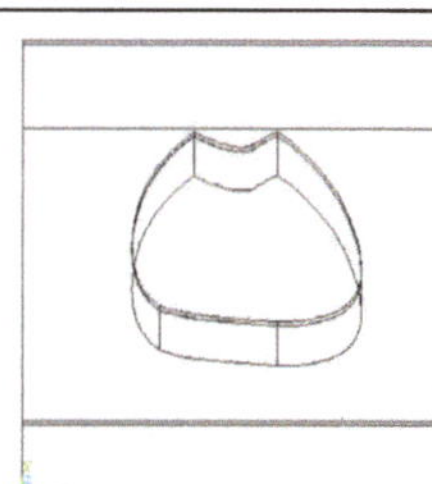

5.2.2 Finite Element Modeling

The accuracy of FEM is significantly affected by both the quality of the meshing and the boundary conditions applied during the simulation process [28–30]. Despite the critical nature of these elements, many computational models developed for wound analysis have neglected to perform a thorough mesh convergence study, which can lead to potential inaccuracies in the results. In a recent investigation conducted by Chanda et al. [31], a comprehensive mesh convergence study was performed utilizing Ansys software. Their goal was to determine the optimal mesh configuration for a computational model that simulates wound closure involving sutures. In the present study, we also conducted a detailed mesh convergence analysis in order to identify the ideal mesh that would enhance the accuracy of stress estimations across various skin-wound models. For this mesh convergence study, we implemented sizing control through elemental division, resulting in the creation of six distinct meshes for the skin-wound model. These meshes varied in granularity: very coarse (comprising 3,564 elements), coarse (7,987 elements), semi-fine (14,881 elements), fine (24,480 elements), very fine (38,154 elements), and superfine (54,834 elements). This range of mesh densities was essential for evaluating how mesh refinement influences the simulation outcomes. In terms of the meshing strategy, the process was initiated with the epidermal layer, as it is the thinnest and most delicate layer of the skin. Following this, the dermal layer was subsequently meshed. This sequential approach was crucial not only for maintaining the integrity of the model but also for ensuring accurate interaction between the two layers, which is vital for the simulation of wound healing processes. By systematically examining these various mesh configurations, we aim to establish a mesh that yields reliable and precise results for future analyses of skin-wound mechanics.

5.2.3 Loads and Boundary Conditions

Human skin is inherently under tension due to its structural composition, and the pre-stress values can fluctuate significantly based on factors such as hydration levels, age, and the specific anatomical site on the body [26, 32, 33]. In the current study, we analyzed the skin pre-stress attributed to this natural tension, focusing on a two-layer skin model that represents both the epidermis and dermis [27]. We applied outward pressure loads of 0.25 kPa and 25 kPa orthogonally to this model to observe how it responds under varying conditions. To ensure the robustness of our simulations, we conducted a mesh convergence study. We maintained a constant pre-stress of $\pm$ 0.25 kPa in the Y-direction while systematically varying the pre-stress values in the X-direction, testing intensities of $\pm$ 10 kPa, $\pm$ 20 kPa, and $\pm$ 30 kPa. Each mesh configuration was carefully evaluated for its maximum von Mises stress, which allowed us to identify the most appropriate mesh for subsequent detailed analyses.

The von Mises stress criterion is widely regarded in material science for its effectiveness in predicting yield or fracture in isotropic and ductile materials when subjected to complex loading conditions. It simplifies the process by calculating overall stresses rather than requiring separate analyses of stresses along each principal direction [34, 35]. In this study, we adopted pre-stress skin values from established literature to ensure our findings align with recognized data [27]. Furthermore, our computational models incorporated a two-layered skin structure, specifically the epidermis and the dermis, along with the associated clot material, which were modeled to be perfectly bonded for the sake of our analysis. We utilized flexible and fully bonded contact pairs to simulate realistic interactions between these materials. To enhance the accuracy of our simulations, we implemented surface-to-surface contact pairs and established an automatic contact adjustment mechanism. This consisted of an initial contact closure factor of five, which was crucial in minimizing penetration between surfaces and ensuring effective gap closure during contact, thereby improving the reliability of our results. This comprehensive approach allowed for a thorough investigation into the mechanical behavior of skin under varying stress conditions.

5.2.4 Material Modeling

The material properties for the skin-wound models were carefully selected from existing literature to accurately represent the average characteristics of the epidermis, dermis, and clot materials involved in wound healing. Specifically, the elastic modulus values were determined to be 1 MPa for the epidermis, which reflects its relatively softer and more flexible nature, 100 MPa for the dermis, denoting its strength and rigidity, and 0.1 MPa for the clot material, indicative of its temporary and supportive role in the healing process. In addition, the Poisson's ratios associated with these materials were recorded as 0.45 for the epidermis, suggesting a high degree of deformation under stress, 0.3 for the dermis, which demonstrates moderate compressibility, and 0.4 for the clot material, indicating its capacity to expand when stretched. The wound healing process was conceptualized in three distinct stages, as depicted in Fig. 5.2. These stages included: the absence of a clot, a partial clot formation of 0.5 mm thickness, and the formation of a complete clot measuring 1 mm. This progressive model allows for a comprehensive understanding of how varying levels of clot formation influence the healing dynamics. To support this analysis, a total of 30 distinct models were developed, which comprised 10 unique wound models each analyzed across the three clot fill stages. This extensive modeling approach enables a thorough computational analysis of the factors influencing wound healing, facilitating insights that could lead to improved medical treatments and interventions.

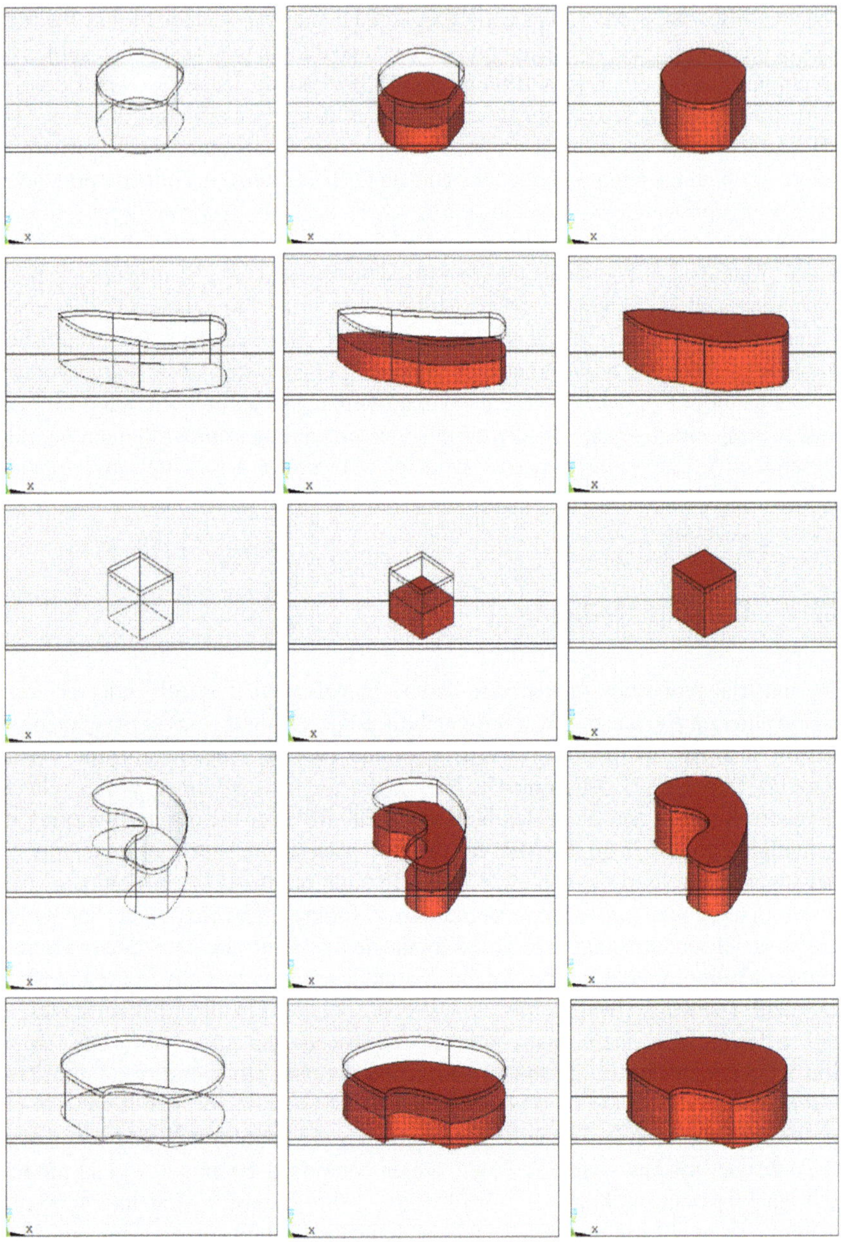

Fig. 5.2 Wound models illustrating the wound healing steps: no clot, half clot, and full clot. *Reproduced under the terms of the Creative Commons Attribution 4.0 International License* [19]

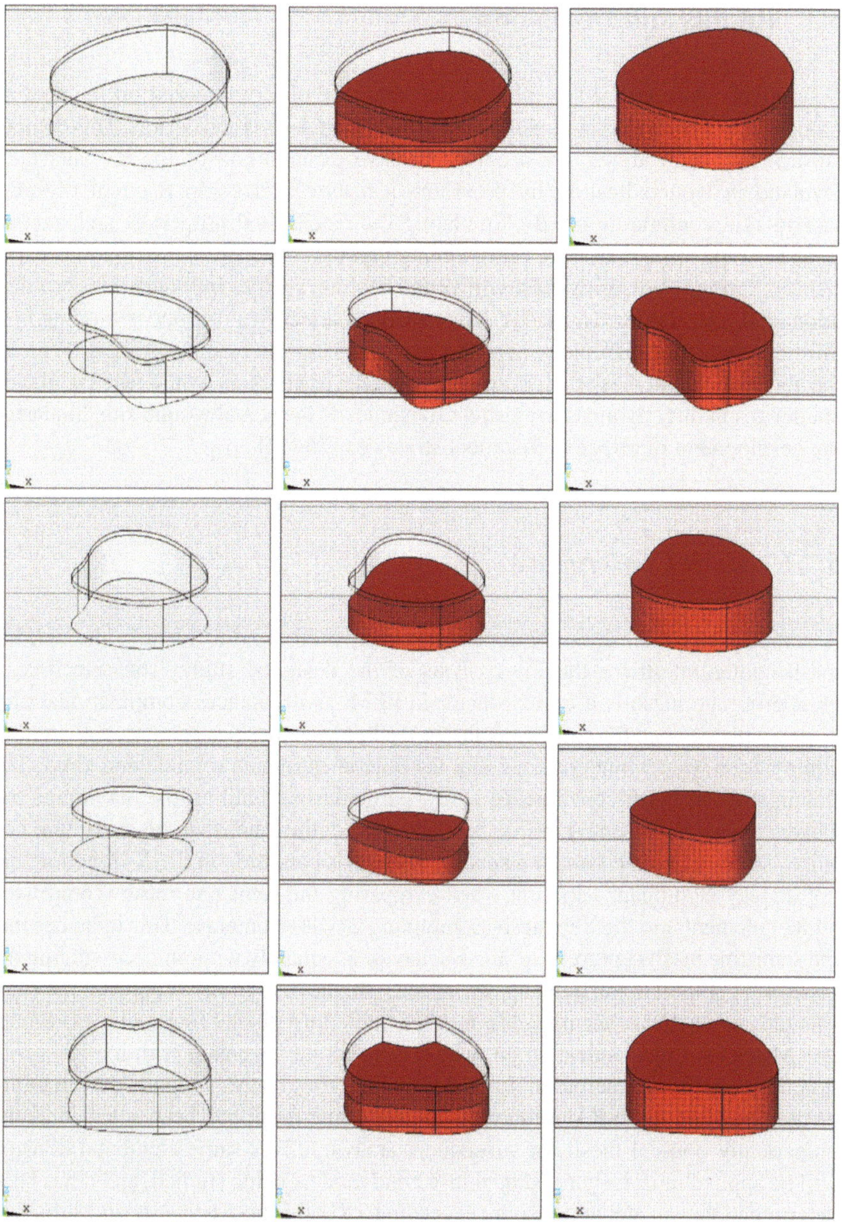

Fig. 5.2 (continued)

5.3 Results and Discussion

(FE models were utilized to analyze the influence of clot material on the healing process of a two-layer skin model, comprising the epidermis and dermis. This computational approach allows for a comprehensive examination of the biomechanics involved in wound healing by providing a macro-level comparison of different wound-skin configurations. By simulating the mechanical properties and interactions between various tissues, FE modeling highlights the stress distributions experienced during the distinct phases of wound healing, such as inflammation, proliferation, and remodeling. These stress distributions are critical for understanding how different materials, like clots, contribute to or hinder the healing process. Without the ability to model these factors computationally, researchers would face significant challenges in directly measuring stress dynamics at the actual wound site, hindering the development of effective treatment strategies [36, 37].

5.3.1 Mesh Convergence

A comprehensive mesh convergence study was performed to identify the optimal mesh configuration for the FE analysis of the designed study. The selection of an appropriate mesh is a critical factor in FEM, as it balances computational efficiency with the need for precise results. A well-chosen mesh can significantly reduce computation time while ensuring that the outcomes remain reliable and valid. The findings of the mesh convergence study, particularly regarding the maximum von Mises stress, are presented in Fig. 5.3. This figure illustrates that the maximum von Mises stress, calculated under a specific pre-stress condition in the X-direction, did not display significant variation when comparing the semi-fine mesh (comprising 14,881 elements) to the fine mesh (comprising 24,480 elements). This indicates that the semi-fine mesh captures the stress behavior adequately without necessitating the increased computational demand associated with the finer mesh. Moreover, the analysis also evaluated other response metrics, including displacement and maximum von Mises total mechanical strain, which were found to remain within a 5% variation. This consistency across multiple response metrics further supports the reliability of the semi-fine mesh. Consequently, the semi-fine mesh has been selected as the numerically optimal mesh for subsequent analyses. This same elemental division will be applied uniformly to other skin-wound models being studied, and it has been determined that an elemental count exceeding 15,000 is both accurate and sufficient to meet the analytical requirements of the project. This approach ensures that the analysis remains both efficient and robust, aligning with best practices in FEM.

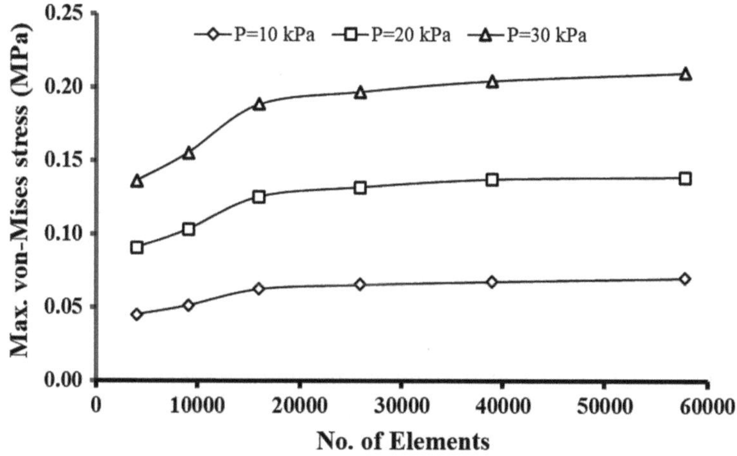

Fig. 5.3 Mesh elements versus maximum von Mises stress in an FE wound model, with 10, 30, and 50 kPa pre-stresses along the X-direction, for mesh convergence study. *Reproduced under the terms of the Creative Commons Attribution 4.0 International License* [19]

5.3.2 Wound Stresses Due to Varying Clot Progression

To gain a comprehensive understanding of stress distribution and the maximum von Mises stress in wound-skin models, we conducted a detailed analysis of all 30 models, which included 10 different wound types evaluated under three clot conditions: no clot, a 0.5 mm clot, and a 1 mm clot. Our findings revealed that the maximum von Mises stress consistently localized at the periphery of the two-layer skin model, with stress values ranging from 140 to 159 kPa across all models. This pattern suggests that the edges of the wound are critical areas where stress concentrations occur, potentially influencing healing and tissue integrity. Further analysis involved comparing the stress values specifically at the wound sites to understand how different geometries of the wounds affect stress distribution. Interestingly, we observed that the stress values at these sites were approximately the same for both the no-clot and clot conditions across all wound types. This indicates that the primary variations in stress may occur within the clot material itself rather than the underlying tissue. Therefore, our results suggest that the characteristics of the clot could play a significant role in stress distribution, which may have implications for treatment approaches in wound management.

At the wound sites, the first group of wounds (wounds 1–3) corresponded to diabetic ulcers, which are known for their challenging healing processes due to impaired blood flow and neuropathy. In this group, the maximum stress concentrations recorded were 96.5 kPa, 93.9 kPa, and 93.4 kPa, respectively. These high stress levels indicate the pressure exerted on the surrounding tissues, which can hinder healing and exacerbate the condition of diabetic wounds. The second group of wounds (wounds 4–6) represented venous ulcers, a common complication related to chronic venous insufficiency. In this category, the wounds showed maximum von Mises stresses of 101.4 kPa, 98.7 kPa, and a notably high 124 kPa, respectively. This elevated stress suggests that the venous wounds are subject to significant mechanical strain, which can impede proper blood circulation and delay recovery. The third group (wounds 7–9) consisted of pressure ulcers, also known as bedsores, which occurred due to excessive pressure on the skin tissue. The maximum stress values recorded at these wound sites were 100.03 kPa, 100.20 kPa, and 96 kPa, respectively. These values reflect the critical role that sustained pressure plays in tissue damage and ulcer formation, particularly in immobile patients. Furthermore, the ulcer wound (wound 10) generated a maximum induced stress of 117.14 kPa at its site. This higher stress level could be attributed to factors such as infection or necrotic tissue, which often complicate ulcer healing. Overall, the findings indicate minimal variations in maximum stress levels across the three types of simulated wounds, highlighting the persistent mechanical challenges faced during the healing process for diabetic, venous, and pressure ulcers. Understanding these stress distributions is crucial for developing targeted treatment strategies that can enhance wound healing and prevent further complications.

5.3.3 Localized Stresses on the Clot for Different Healing Phases

The study focused on the induced stresses acting on the clot material during the healing process. Our analysis revealed that the maximum von Mises stress values exhibited a significant reduction across all analyzed wound cases for both healing phases, specifically at clot thicknesses of 0.5 mm and 1 mm. This decrease in stress suggests an improvement in the structural integrity of the clot as it progresses through different stages of healing, indicating a more favorable environment for tissue regeneration.

Localized Induced Stresses for 0.5 mm Clot Material

Figure 5.4 presents the von Mises stress distribution across wounds (1–10) that were treated with a 0.5 mm layer of clot material. In the case of wound 1, the analysis revealed that the maximum stress at the wound site measured 0.12 kPa. This value is significantly lower than the stress experienced by an open wound, which was recorded at 96.5 kPa. This drastic reduction in stress suggests that the application of the clot material could facilitate a more expedited healing process for this specific wound configuration. For wound 2, the maximum stress recorded was slightly lower at 0.082 kPa, occurring at a corner along the top layer of the clot. Similar to wound 1, this indicates local stress concentration, while the majority of the clot's surface exhibited healing under very low stress, showing variations from 0.02 to 0.06 kPa. This suggests that the clot effectively distributes stress away from the wound area, promoting a conducive environment for healing. In the case of wound 3, the maximum stress observed at the wound site was approximately 0.14 kPa. Although this is a higher value compared to the previous wounds, it still remains significantly lower than that observed in an open wound. The stress distribution within this wound was fairly uniform; the maximum stress recorded at the side of the clot attached to the wound was a mere 0.03 kPa. In contrast, the top layer of the clot showed a range of stress values between 0.04 and 0.14 kPa. This variability highlights the complex interaction between the clot and the underlying tissue, suggesting that while some areas of the clot may experience stress, the overall mechanism remains effective in promoting healing. Overall, the data underscores the potential benefits of using clot material in wound treatment, indicating that it not only reduces stress on the wound site but also contributes to a favorable healing environment.

In the assessment of venous wounds classified as wounds 4–6, significant reductions in stress at the wound sites were observed when clot material was applied. For example, in wound 4, the initial maximum stress measured at the wound site was 101.4 kPa; however, this was significantly decreased to just 0.17 kPa upon applying a 0.5 mm thick clot. This substantial reduction highlights the effectiveness of the clot in distributing mechanical stress away from the vulnerable tissue. In the case of wound 5, the analysis revealed that the maximum stress at the edge of the clot, oriented in the direction of the applied pressure, peaked at 0.12 kPa. The stress distribution across the surface of the clot was found to be relatively uniform, ranging from 0.23 kPa down to 0.08 kPa. This is particularly noteworthy, as it represents a significant reduction compared to the stress levels recorded in the open wound, which stood at 98.7 kPa. Such a drastic difference underscores the protective advantage provided by the clot in managing physiological stresses during the healing process. For wound 6, the maximum stress recorded was 0.18 kPa, occurring at a specific point along the side thickness of the 0.5 mm clot. This finding is pertinent as it indicates that

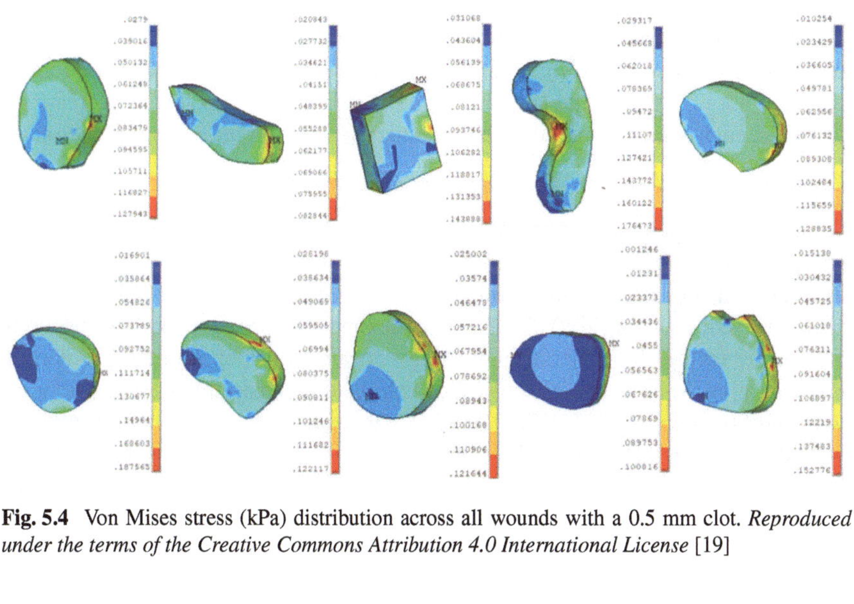

Fig. 5.4 Von Mises stress (kPa) distribution across all wounds with a 0.5 mm clot. *Reproduced under the terms of the Creative Commons Attribution 4.0 International License* [19]

even small variations in clot thickness can influence localized stress concentrations. Overall, the presence of the clot material not only reduces mechanical stress at the wound sites but also plays a crucial role in facilitating the healing process by minimizing stress concentration, thereby promoting a more conducive environment for tissue repair.

The next category of wounds examined consisted of pressure wounds (wounds 7–9) and ulcer wounds (wound 10), each displaying distinct characteristics and stress responses. In wound 7, the analysis revealed that a clot measuring 0.5 mm in thickness experienced a maximum stress of 0.12 kPa at its thickest point. Notably, as the distance increased from the point of applied pressure, the stresses within the clot diminished significantly. This resulted in a uniform distribution of stress across the clot layer and on the side of the clot attached to the wound bed, indicating an effective pressure management within the healing tissue. Wound 8 exhibited the same maximum stress of 0.12 kPa at the 0.5 mm clot; however, this value was strikingly lower compared to that of an open wound, which recorded a maximum stress of 100.20 kPa. The significant difference underscores the effectiveness of clot formation in mitigating stress compared to an unprotected wound environment. For wound 9, the analysis showed that the maximum von Mises stress at the clot, also 0.5 mm thick, was 0.10 kPa. This stress was localized at the corner of the wound, where pressure typically magnifies. Like the previous wounds, it was observed that stress was evenly distributed across the surface of the clot, remaining substantially lower than the stress levels associated with the open wound, which measured 96 kPa. This consistently lower stress indicates that the clot may protect surrounding tissues from excessive pressure. In the case of wound 10, which presented as an ulcer, it was determined that the unique shape and characteristics of the wound could facilitate a more straightforward healing process without placing significant stress on the underlying skin surface. In this instance, the 0.5 mm clot displayed a stress value of 0.15 kPa at the corner closest to the applied pressure. Just as in the other wounds, the stress distribution was even across the clot surface, markedly lower than the 117.14 kPa observed in the corresponding open wound. This pattern suggests that the formed clot may not only contribute to hemostasis but also play a pivotal role in creating a favorable environment for healing by minimizing stress on the surrounding tissues.

Localized Induced Stresses for 1 mm Clot Material

Figure 5.5 provides a detailed representation of the von Mises stress distribution across various wound sites with a clot thickness of 1 mm. In wound 1, when the clot thickness was increased from 0.5 mm to 1 mm, a significant decrease in stress value was observed, dropping to 0.09 kPa. The maximum stress concentration occurred at a corner of the clot material, indicating a localized response to the mechanical forces at play. Most of the clot's surface exhibited a consistent stress distribution, with values ranging from 0.02 to 0.48 kPa on the side of the clot in contact with the wound, while the top layer of the clot presented lower stress values, ranging from 0.05 to 0.09 kPa. This demonstrates that the attachment surface is subject to higher stress concentrations compared to the upper region of the clot. In the case of wound 2, a 1 mm clot showed a maximum stress value of 0.78 kPa, again occurring at a corner of the clot. The stress distribution in this scenario was comparable to that observed with a 0.5 mm clot, suggesting that despite the increase in thickness, the stress dynamics remained relatively consistent. For wound 3, however, the maximum stress value for the 1 mm clot was reduced to 0.12 kPa, located at the center of the clot. This reduction in maximum stress indicates a change in the mechanical response as the pressure was applied. Additionally, this value represents a 16% decrease in maximum stress compared to the 0.5 mm clot, signaling a potential improvement in stress distribution with the thicker clot material, which might contribute to better wound healing outcomes by reducing peak stresses that could lead to tissue damage. The propagation of stress in the direction of the applied pressure further illustrates the mechanical behavior of the clot, highlighting the importance of understanding these dynamics in wound treatment and management.

In the analysis of venous wounds (wounds 4–6), significant variations in stress distribution and concentration were observed with changes in clot thickness. For wound 4, the maximum stress value reached 0.26 kPa, which was detected specifically at a corner of the 1 mm clot. This localized increase in stress suggests a heightened risk of further complications in that area. The overall distribution of stress values across the clot's surface ranged between 0.16 kPa and 0.02 kPa, indicating a pronounced gradient that diminished in areas further from the direction of applied pressure. Notably, the region exhibiting maximum stress concentration was considerably smaller in the 1 mm clot compared to the 0.5 mm clot, which may correlate with better mechanical stability and reduced risk of wound dehiscence. In wound 5, the initial stress value of 0.12 kPa was further reduced to 0.10 kPa with the application of 1 mm of clotting thickness. This reduction in stress underscores the role of increased clot thickness in mitigating stress concentration, which can significantly aid in wound

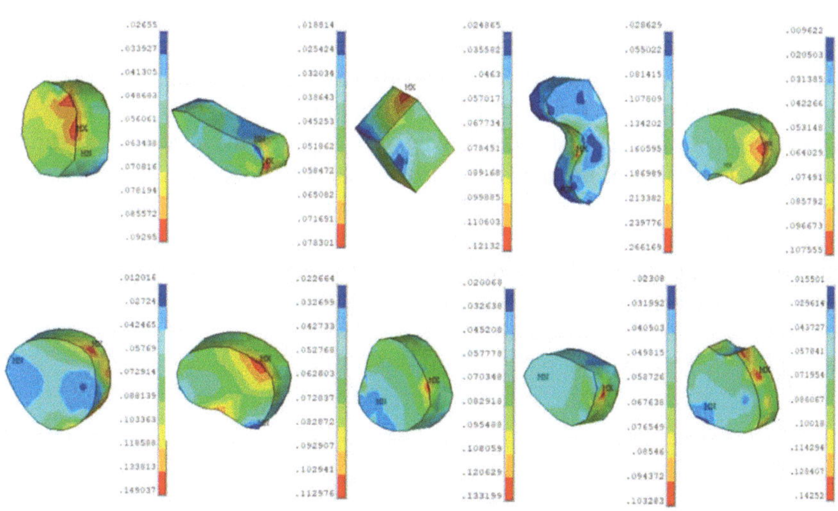

Fig. 5.5 Stress distribution (kPa) across all wounds with a 1 mm clot. *Reproduced under the terms of the Creative Commons Attribution 4.0 International License* [19]

healing. The larger clot thickness contributed to a dramatic 17% decrease in overall stress concentration, facilitating a more conducive environment for tissue repair. Wound 6 presented a maximum stress value of 0.14 kPa, noted at both the corners and within the thickness of the 1 mm clot. In contrast, the maximum stress value observed in the 0.5 mm clot was 0.18 kPa, illustrating a reduction as the clot thickness increased to 1 mm. The stress distribution patterns for wound 6 were largely analogous to those seen in the thinner clot, hinting at similar healing dynamics. This consistency in stress responses across different clot thicknesses underscores the potential for enhanced healing timelines associated with greater clot thickness. Overall, the findings indicate that increasing the thickness of the clot significantly affects stress distribution, promoting favorable healing conditions and minimizing the risk of complications.

In wound 7, the analysis of stress distribution revealed that a 1 mm clot exhibited a maximum stress value of 0.11 kPa, which is comparable to the 0.5 mm clot that reached 0.12 kPa. This similarity indicates that the presence of the clot plays a significant role in promoting stress-free healing, as it effectively reduces the pressure on the wound when contrasted with an open wound scenario, where the maximum stress was alarmingly high at 100 kPa. For wound 8, an increase in clot thickness to 1 mm resulted in a localized stress value of 0.13 kPa at a particular point within the wound clot. The other sections of the clot maintained stress distribution patterns akin to those observed in the 0.5 mm clot. This wound configuration suggests an enhanced healing potential, allowing for a more rapid recovery due to the reduced mechanical stress placed on the healing tissue. In wound 9, we found that the maximum stress recorded was 0.10 kPa, occurring at a small region of the 1 mm clot, which closely parallels the maximum stress value seen in the 0.5 mm clot. The majority of the clot's surface demonstrated a uniform distribution of stresses within the range of 0.02 to 0.07 kPa, providing an optimal environment for healing by minimizing excessive pressure on the wound. Turning to wound 10, the stress value observed was slightly higher at 0.14 kPa, but this was still confined to a small area of the 1 mm clot. The bulk of the clot continued to exhibit stress values ranging from 0.01 to 0.10 kPa. This low-stress distribution is encouraging, as it supports the necessary conditions for adequate healing of the ulcerated wound, facilitating the body's natural repair processes without undue strain on the surrounding tissues. Overall, the findings emphasize the crucial role of clot thickness in managing wound stress, with thicker clots providing better conditions for healing by maintaining lower stress levels and promoting an environment conducive to recovery.

5.4 Comparative Analysis of the Wound Geometry and Clot Filling

The analysis of wound healing across various skin-wound models was conducted to evaluate the effects of different clot thicknesses, specifically focusing on two stages of clot filling: a half clot measuring 0.5 mm and a full clot measuring 1 mm. This assessment was compared against an open wound scenario, which lacked any clotting material. The details of this comparative analysis, particularly the maximal von Mises stress for each wound case, are presented in Table 5.2. The results indicated a pronounced reduction in stress concentration due to the presence of clot material, demonstrating a decrease of over 99% when compared to the stress values observed in open wounds across all examined cases. This significant reduction not only highlights the mechanical advantages of clot formation but also underscores its role in promoting more effective wound healing. Interestingly, the findings reveal that the full clot (1 mm) exhibited a more pronounced capability in reducing stress levels than the half clot (0.5 mm), as evidenced by the majority of wound cases studied. However, exceptions were noted in wounds 4 and 8, where the differences were less pronounced. It is worth mentioning that even in these two instances, the highest stress concentration was localized solely at the edges of the clot material, suggesting that the central regions of the clot still facilitated an environment conducive to healing. Overall, the results indicate that regardless of the wound's geometry or clot thickness, whether 0.5 mm or 1 mm, the initiation of clot formation plays a crucial role in accelerating the healing process of skin wounds. The presence of clot material not only promotes uniform stress distribution but also supports quicker recovery, further emphasizing its importance in the wound healing process.

Figure 5.6 provides a detailed comparison of the maximum induced stress levels at the wound site when using two different clot material thicknesses: 0.5 mm and 1 mm,

Table 5.2 Decrease in the Max. von Mises stress with clot. *Reproduced under the terms of the Creative Commons Attribution 4.0 International License* [19]

Wound No	Max. von mises stress (kPa)		
	No clot (Open wound)	0.5 mm clot	1 mm clot
wound 1	96.5206	0.12794	0.09295
wound 2	93.9234	0.08284	0.07830
wound 3	93.4778	0.14389	0.12132
wound 4	101.4920	0.17647	0.26617
wound 5	98.7476	0.12884	0.10756
wound 6	124.0500	0.18757	0.14904
wound 7	100.0330	0.12212	0.11298
wound 8	100.2070	0.12164	0.13320
wound 9	96.0096	0.10082	0.10328
wound 10	117.1410	0.15278	0.14252

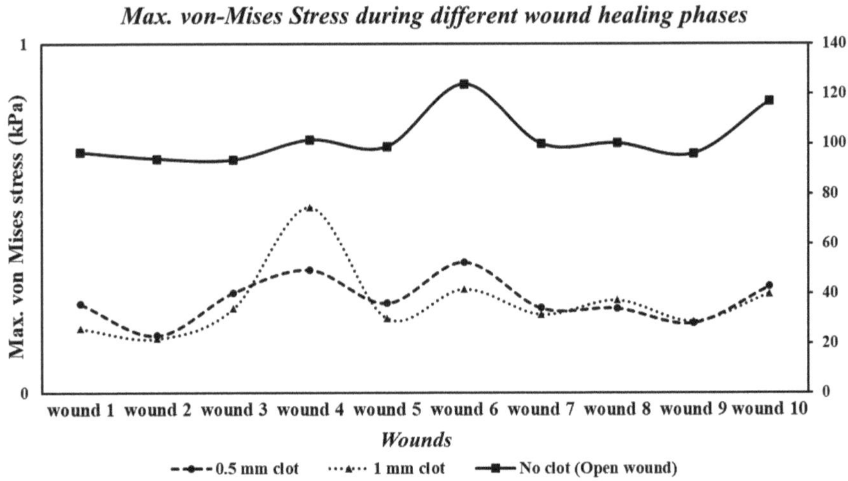

Fig. 5.6 Comparative plot for stress concentration at different clot stages. *Reproduced under the terms of the Creative Commons Attribution 4.0 International License* [19]

in contrast to an open wound without any clot. The data demonstrate a clear trend: as the wound progresses towards healing, the stress concentration around the area decreases. This reduction in stress reaches its most significant point once the clot has fully formed at a thickness of 1 mm. In the analysis of wound 4, the maximum von Mises stress was particularly notable at the edge of the clot's thickness. This localized increase in stress serves to highlight the complexities involved in wound healing; the thicker 1 mm clot produced a greater stress response compared to the thinner 0.5 mm clot. For wounds 7 through 10, the findings indicated that there was minimal change in stress distribution as the clot developed further. This suggests that once a certain threshold of clot material is reached, additional layers may not significantly alter the stress dynamics. Overall, this analysis leads to the critical conclusion that both clot thicknesses, whether 0.5 mm or 1 mm, substantially reduce the stress concentration in comparison to an unprotected open wound. This reduction is beneficial as it facilitates timely healing and plays a crucial role in preventing bacterial pathogens from directly adhering to the wound surface, thereby reducing the risk of infection and promoting an optimal healing environment.

5.5 Conclusions

This study investigates the complex mechanics of wounded and healing skin through the use of FEM, a computational technique that allows for detailed simulations of physical phenomena. A novel computational model was developed, taking into account the realistic shapes and sizes of wounds as reported in the scientific literature. The research specifically examines the stresses that arise during the wound healing process, focusing on three distinct phases: the initial phase of an open wound with no clotting, a transitional phase with a partial clot measuring 0.5 mm, and a final phase featuring a fully formed clot measuring 1 mm. By analyzing these different stages, the study aims to uncover the mechanical behavior of the skin as it undergoes healing. Understanding the dynamics of wound healing is crucial, as it can significantly contribute to the advancement of medical treatments, healing solutions, and surgical procedures. By employing this computational model, researchers hope to enhance our knowledge of the healing process, ultimately leading to better patient outcomes and innovative approaches in wound care.

The results of the study revealed that the formation of clot material during the healing process significantly mitigated localized deformations and stress concentrations in the surrounding skin. As the clot developed, the maximum stress levels at the wound sites experienced a substantial reduction of up to 89%. This reduction highlights the protective role of clot material in wound healing. Furthermore, the maximum stresses observed at the clot material were astonishingly up to 99% lower than those found in cases of open wounds. This drastic decrease emphasizes the effectiveness of clot formation in maintaining tissue integrity and reducing strain on damaged areas. Additionally, a notable decline in stress concentration was recorded at the clot material during the clotting phase, indicating that the presence of the clot provides enhanced support compared to the unprotected state of an open wound. Interestingly, the study found that the stress distribution within the clot material remained relatively stable, showing minimal variability with changes in wound size and skin pre-stress. The only significant alterations observed were associated with the shape of the wound itself, suggesting that while external factors like wound dimensions influence healing, the clot material effectively stabilizes stress within the wound environment. This highlights the critical role of clot formation in the wound healing process and its importance in managing stress distribution across injured tissues.

References

1. Chanda A, Upchurch W (2018) Biomechanical modeling of wounded skin. J Compos Sci 2, Page 69
2. Chanda A (2018) Biomechanical modeling of human skin tissue surrogates. Biomimetics 3, Page 18
3. Chanda A, Unnikrishnan V, Lackey K, Robbins J (2019) Biofidelic conductive soft tissue surrogates 69, 127–135. https://doi.org/10.1080/00914037.2018.1552856
4. Lapeer RJ, Gasson PD, Karri V (2011) A hyperelastic finite-element model of human skin for interactive real-time surgical simulation. IEEE Trans Biomed Eng 58:1013–1022
5. Singh G, Chanda A (2021) Mechanical properties of whole-body soft human tissues : a review. Biomed Mater 16:062004
6. Makode S, Singh G, Chanda A (2021) Development of novel anisotropic skin simulants. Phys Scr 96:125019
7. Singh G, Gupta V, Chanda A (2022) Artificial skin with varying biomechanical properties. Mater. Today Proc. 62:3162–3166
8. Rostami B et al (2021) Multiclass wound image classification using an ensemble deep CNN-based classifier. Comput Biol Med 134:104536

9. Marijanović D, Filko D (2020) A systematic overview of recent methods for non-contact chronic wound analysis. Appl. Sci. 10, Page 7613
10. Stillman RM, Bella FJ, Seligman SJ (1980) Skin wound closure: the effect of various wound closure methods on susceptibility to infection. Arch Surg 115:674–675
11. Flynn C (2010) Finite element models of wound closure. J Tissue Viability 19:137–149
12. Cumming BD, McElwain DLS, Upton Z (2009) A mathematical model of wound healing and subsequent scarring. J R Soc Interface 7:19–34
13. Baum CL, Arpey CJ (2006) Normal cutaneous wound healing: clinical correlation with cellular and molecular events. Dermatologic Surg 31:674–686
14. Janes LE et al (2020) Modeling tissue expansion with isogeometric analysis: Skin growth and tissue level changes in the porcine model. Plast Reconstr Surg 792–798 https://doi.org/10.1097/PRS.0000000000007153
15. Kim MH et al (2008) Dynamics of neutrophil infiltration during cutaneous wound healing and infection using fluorescence imaging. J Invest Dermatol 128:1812–1820
16. Lynch SE, Colvin RB, Antoniades HN (1989) Growth factors in wound healing. Single and synergistic effects on partial thickness porcine skin wounds. J Clin Invest 84, 640–646
17. Van Zuijlen PPM et al (2003) Collagen morphology in human skin and scar tissue: No adaptations in response to mechanical loading at joints. Burns 29:423–431
18. Verhaegen PDHM et al (2009) Differences in collagen architecture between keloid, hypertrophic scar, normotrophic scar, and normal skin: An objective histopathological analysis. Wound Repair Regen. 17:649–656
19. Singh G, Chanda A (2022) Biomechanical modeling of progressive wound healing: A computational study. Biomed Eng Adv. 4:100055
20. Flynn C, McCormack BAO (2008) A simplified model of scar contraction. J Biomech 41:1582–1589
21. Thomson GA (2007) An investigation of leakage tracts along stressed suture lines in phantom tissue. Med Eng Phys 29:1030–1034
22. Singh G, Gupta S, Chanda A (2021) Biomechanical modelling of diabetic foot ulcers: A computational study. J Biomech 127:110699
23. Gupta S, Gupta V, Chanda A (2022) Biomechanical modeling of novel high expansion auxetic skin grafts. Int J Numer Method Biomed Eng. e3586 https://doi.org/10.1002/CNM.3586
24. Larrabee WF, Galt JA (1986) A finite element model of skin deformation. III. the finite element model. Laryngoscope 96:413–419
25. Cavicchi A, Gambarotta L, Massabò R (2009) Computational modeling of reconstructive surgery: The effects of the natural tension on skin wrinkling. Finite Elem Anal Des 45:519–529
26. Capek L, Jacquet E, Dzan L, Simunek A (2012) The analysis of forces needed for the suturing of elliptical skin wounds. Med Biol Eng Comput 50:193–198
27. Chanda A, Unnikrishnan V (2017) A realistic 3D computational model of the closure of skin wound with interrupted sutures. J Mech Med Biol 17
28. Gupta V, Chanda A (2022) Biomechanics of skin grafts: effect of pattern size, spacing and orientation. Eng Res Express 4:015006
29. Gupta V, Chanda A (2022) Expansion potential of skin grafts with alternating slit based auxetic incisions. Forces Mech. 7:100092
30. Gupta S, Singh G, Chanda A (2021) Prediction of diabetic foot ulcer progression: a computational study. Biomed Phys Eng Express 7:065020
31. Chanda A, Unnikrishnan V, Richter HE, Lockhart ME (2016) A biofidelic computational model of the female pelvic system to understand effect of bladder fill and progressive vaginal tissue stiffening due to prolapse on anterior vaginal wall. Int J Numer Method Biomed Eng. 32:e02767
32. Chanda A, Unnikrishnan V, Lackey K (2017) Biofidelic conductive synthetic skin composites. In: 32nd technical conference of the american society for composites 1 400–408 (DEStech Publications Inc., 2017)
33. Gupta V, Singh G, Chanda A (2023) Modeling of metamaterial based incision patterns for generating high expansions in skin grafts. Clin Biomech 110:106118

34. Zhang M, Zheng YP, Mak AFT (1997) Estimating the effective Young's modulus of soft tissues from indentation tests—nonlinear finite element analysis of effects of friction and large deformation. Med Eng Phys 19:512–517
35. Xie H, Song J, Zhong Y, Gu C (2020) Kalman filter finite element method for real-time soft tissue modeling. IEEE Access 8:53471–53483
36. Singh G, Chanda A (2024) Finite element modeling of diabetic foot: a state-of-the-art review. Eng. Res. Express 6:012507
37. Levy A, Frank MBO, Gefen A (2015) The biomechanical efficacy of dressings in preventing heel ulcers. J Tissue Viability 24:1–11

Chapter 6
Literature on Management of Diabetic Foot Ulcers

6.1 Introduction

Diabetic foot ulcers (DFUs) are a significant and pressing health concern that requires significant attention, management, and treatment. The formation of these ulcers among diabetic patients is influenced by various critical factors, including the ulcer's depth, its specific anatomical location, and the presence of ischemia, defined as a reduction in blood supply to the affected area. Plantar ulcers, which are located on the underside of the foot, often impact vital regions such as the forefoot, midfoot, and hindfoot. These locations are particularly susceptible to injury and pressure, given the weight-bearing nature of the foot. In contrast, non-plantar ulcers typically manifest on the dorsal (top) surface of the foot, which can also be prone to trauma but may have different healing dynamics and risk factors [1, 2]. Statistics reveal a concerning fact that approximately 68% of DFUs are classified as superficial, indicating that they affect only the outer layers of skin. However, more severe cases exist, with around 15% of these ulcers penetrating down to the tendons and an additional 17% involving the bone. This wide spectrum of ulcer severity underscores the importance of early detection and intervention in order to prevent complications. According to recent studies, about 65% of DFUs achieve complete healing within a designated period, which can vary depending on individual circumstances and treatment adherence [3, 4].

Unfortunately, the reality remains that 16% of ulcers fail to heal, presenting a considerable challenge in the field of diabetic foot care. This stagnant healing can result in extended periods of discomfort and significantly impair the quality of life for patients. More alarmingly, the consequences of untreated foot ulcers can be dire. Statistics show that approximately 15.5% of DFUs lead to lower limb amputations due to complications such as severe infections or gangrene [5]. Moreover, 3.5% of affected patients experience mortality attributed to their ulcerative conditions, underscoring the critical need for effective management strategies. Ulcers can also be classified based on their duration, which has a direct impact on treatment

A. Chanda and G. Singh, *Diabetic Foot Ulcer*, Biomedical Materials for Multi-functional Applications, https://doi.org/10.1007/978-981-95-2484-6_6

approaches. Acute ulcers are defined as those lasting up to 2 weeks, requiring immediate care focused on wound healing. Subacute ulcers persist between 2 and 8 weeks and may necessitate more extensive intervention. Persistent ulcers, lasting longer than 2 months, typically require comprehensive management plans that address not only the wound itself but also underlying issues such as blood flow and infection. Evaluating ulcer size involves careful consideration of both surface area and depth; accurately assessing depth can be particularly challenging but is crucial for determining the appropriate treatment. Various methods, including measuring devices and imaging techniques, may be utilized to aid this assessment [2, 6].

Among the various complications commonly associated with diabetic foot health is flatfoot, a condition characterized by the collapse of the foot's arch. This may cause the entire plantar surface to come into prolonged contact with the ground during standing or movement, leading to an array of complications. Flatfoot can result from several factors, including genetic predisposition, excessive wear on plantar structures, weakened foot arches, or prior injuries. Notably, the prevalence of flatfoot is higher among individuals who are overweight, as excess weight can place additional stress on the foot's structures [7]. Complications arising from flatfoot often stem from the excessive stretching of the Achilles tendon and supportive ligaments, which can lead to discomfort and further musculoskeletal issues. The altered biomechanics associated with flatfoot can create uneven load distributions during ambulation, resulting in excessive supination (rolling outward) and pronation (rolling inward). These mechanical imbalances can not only exacerbate existing diabetic foot problems but also hinder their effective management [8]. A comprehensive understanding of these multifaceted aspects of DFUs and their associated conditions allows healthcare providers to enhance their ability to assist patients in preventing complications and promoting effective healing strategies. Proactive management and awareness of factors contributing to diabetic foot health are crucial in improving patient outcomes and the overall quality of life for individuals living with diabetes.

One of the primary risk factors for the development of plantar ulcers in diabetic individuals is excessive foot pressure. This pressure can result from improper footwear, foot deformities, or other biomechanical issues. In response, healthcare providers often recommend a range of interventions designed to reduce plantar pressure, which may include orthotic devices, specialized footwear, and behavioral modifications to promote better foot care practices. In summary, DFUs are a complex condition influenced by a myriad of factors that require holistic and proactive management strategies to enhance healing outcomes and prevent serious complications. Understanding the nuances of ulcer classification, assessment, and treatment is vital for healthcare providers, patients, and caregivers alike.

A widely recognized and effective strategy for managing diabetic foot health is the use of custom insoles specifically designed to relieve pressure on high-risk areas of the foot. Research has shown that these insoles can significantly reduce the incidence of foot ulcers by redistributing pressure and providing better support. Furthermore, impaired blood circulation is a critical factor contributing to diabetic foot pain and the development of ulcers. Studies indicate that around 60–70% of individuals living with diabetes experience neuropathy, leading to nerve damage [9].

This damage can compromise an individual's ability to feel pain or discomfort, which significantly heightens the risk of ulcer formation, as minor injuries can go unnoticed and untreated. Additional factors exacerbating the risk of ulceration include poorly fitting footwear and existing foot deformities, such as bunions or hammertoes. These conditions can create increased pressure points on the foot, thereby accelerating the onset of diabetic ulcers [10, 11]. It is essential to prioritize proper footwear that accommodates the unique shape and needs of the diabetic foot to mitigate these risks. Interestingly, research has shown that demographic factors such as sex and the specific ulcer site, be it on the forefoot, midfoot, or hindfoot, do not have a significant impact on the healing time of ulcers. This insight underscores the importance of focusing treatment strategies on individual patient factors, including their overall health, preexisting comorbidities, and personal medical histories, rather than relying exclusively on demographic information [5].

Conservative orthotic care plays a crucial role in the management of foot ulcers by off-loading pressure from the affected area, enabling patients to maintain a degree of mobility. These specialized orthotic devices are designed to significantly reduce plantar pressure, which alleviates stress on the ulcerated tissue and promotes the healing process (see Fig. 6.1). The primary objective of this medical intervention is to redistribute the pressure that affects the plantar fascia, a critical area often implicated in the development of foot ulcers. To achieve optimal results, a diverse range of materials, each varying in density, cushioning properties, and shock absorption capabilities, can be employed in the fabrication of foot orthoses. This flexibility allows for a high degree of customization tailored to each patient's individual needs and foot morphology. Unlike prefabricated orthotics, which may not conform perfectly to the unique shape of the foot, custom foot orthoses offer enhanced therapeutic benefits by ensuring full contact with the plantar surface. This comprehensive fit not only improves comfort but also maximizes support and stability, thereby facilitating better weight distribution and reducing the risk of further ulceration [12, 13]. Overall, the use of tailored orthotic devices is a vital strategy in managing and healing foot ulcers, ultimately enhancing the patient's quality of life and promoting a return to normal activities.

6.2 Effect of Diabetes on the Foot

Diabetes can significantly impact foot health due to various physiological changes. One of the primary effects of diabetes is skin dryness coupled with a decreased sense of sensation, known as peripheral neuropathy. These conditions negatively affect both the structure and function of the foot, making it more vulnerable to injuries. Moreover, diabetes often leads to fluctuations in foot pressure distribution. This variation creates areas of high pressure on the foot, particularly in those regions that are subjected to repeated stress, which can lead to the development of neuropathic ulcers [15–18]. To better understand these changes, researchers have utilized advanced techniques such as finite element analysis and magnetic resonance imaging (MRI). These

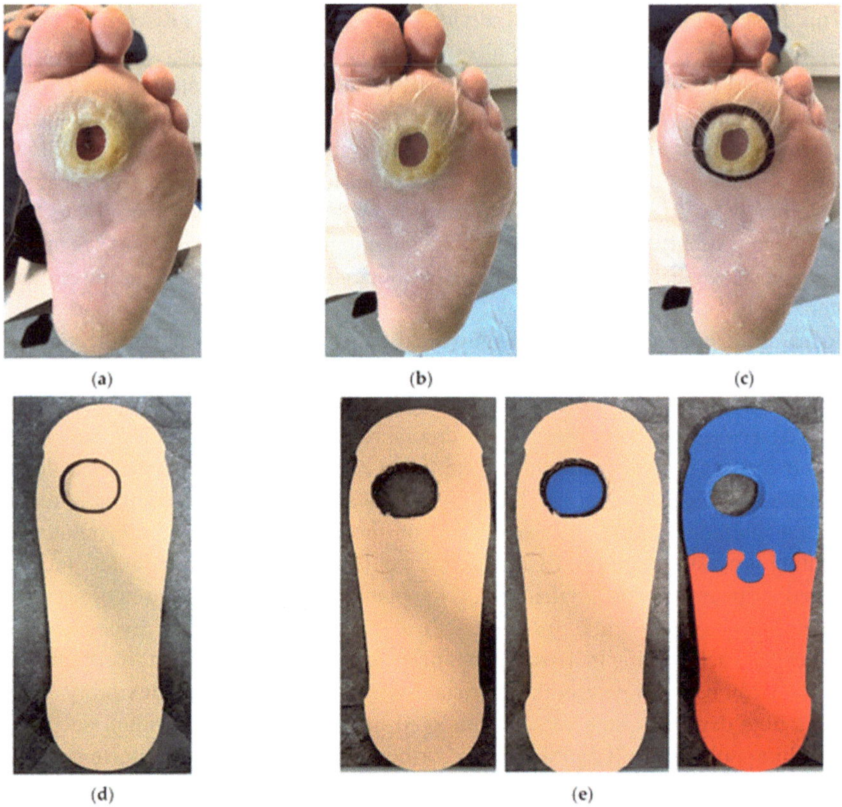

Fig. 6.1 Personalization of the removable cast walker (RCW) insole: **a** DFU localization; **b** Application of transparent sterile dressing; **c** DFU is marked on the transparent sterile dressing; **d** Imprinting of the DFU contour on the mid-layer of the RCW insole; **e** A cone-shaped cut-off is performed in the mid and deep layer of the RCW insole to off-load the DFU area. *Reproduced under the terms of the Creative Commons Attribution 4.0 International License* [14]

studies have revealed a significant increase in the stiffness of the plantar tissue in individuals with diabetes. The results indicate not only a decrease in skin hardness and tissue thickness but also suggest that the diabetic plantar tissue exhibits higher shear and elastic moduli, which could facilitate the formation of ulcers in sensitive areas. Furthermore, diabetes may result in reduced joint mobility in the ankle and foot, leading to abnormal patterns of foot pressure [19]. This lack of mobility can exacerbate the development of high-pressure zones, increasing the susceptibility to ulcers. The presence of foot ulcers is the most common reason for amputations among diabetic patients and often leads to serious complications, including infections and increased morbidity [20]. Alarmingly, the recurrence rate of these ulcers is quite high, even after appropriate treatment has been provided. Research indicates that about 40% of DFUs occur in the plantar zone, particularly near the metatarsal heads, which are regions that endure significant weight-bearing pressure.

The lack of sensory feedback in these areas contributes to an irregular weight-bearing gait, which in turn amplifies forces on the foot and elevates plantar pressure, creating a cycle that further increases the risk of ulceration. Given these complexities, patient education becomes a vital component of managing foot health in individuals with diabetes [21]. Educating patients about essential foot care practices, such as daily inspections for injuries, proper hygiene, and the importance of well-fitting footwear, is crucial. Additionally, teaching adequate wound care techniques can help prevent complications and improve outcomes. By emphasizing preventive measures and regular foot assessments, it is possible to reduce the likelihood of ulcer formation and the associated risks of severe complications [22].

6.3 Different Types of Foot Orthoses

Foot orthoses, commonly referred to as orthotic insoles or arch supports, are specially designed devices that cover the plantar region of the foot, playing a crucial role in providing support for weight-bearing activities such as walking, running, and standing. To achieve optimal effectiveness, these orthoses must be accurately positioned just beneath the foot, ensuring proper alignment and support during movement [23]. The classification of foot orthoses primarily depends on the materials utilized in their fabrication, which significantly influence their characteristics, including stiffness and flexibility. Different materials yield varying levels of support based on individual patient needs and conditions. Key factors that determine the performance of these orthoses include density, thickness, and compression set, all of which affect the overall flexibility or rigidity of the device. In terms of functionality, foot orthoses can be categorized into three main types: accommodating, corrective, and supporting. Accommodating orthoses are designed to distribute pressure evenly across the foot, providing relief for individuals with conditions such as diabetes or arthritis. Corrective orthoses aim to address specific biomechanical issues, such as overpronation or supination, to promote better alignment and foot function. Supporting orthoses, on the other hand, are intended to provide enhanced arch support and stability for individuals engaged in high-impact activities or those requiring additional balance [24]. Furthermore, the classification of foot orthoses is also influenced by the material properties. They can be divided into three categories: soft, semirigid, and hard. Soft orthoses are often made from foam or gel materials to offer maximum cushioning and comfort. Semirigid orthoses strike a balance between support and flexibility, making them suitable for a wide range of activities. Hard orthoses, typically constructed from rigid plastic or carbon fiber, provide firm support and correction for more pronounced foot abnormalities. Understanding these classifications and their specific applications is crucial for selecting the most appropriate orthotic solution tailored to individual patient needs.

Among the various types of orthotic devices available, accommodating foot orthoses are particularly prevalent due to their specific function of reducing stress and strain on the prominent areas of the foot. These orthoses are typically constructed using soft, low-density materials, which allow for a cushioning effect that alleviates discomfort and pressure during daily activities [25]. In contrast, supporting and corrective orthoses are essential for maintaining the structural integrity of the lower extremities. These orthoses function primarily during the stance phase of walking or standing by counteracting the ground reaction forces that can cause abnormal motion in the skeleton. By effectively managing over-pronation, these devices regulate the movements of the subtalar and metatarsal joints, thereby promoting proper alignment and reducing the risk of injury [26]. Semirigid orthoses play a dual role in foot support, combining the protective and cushioning qualities needed to manage foot stress. They typically feature a cushioned top layer designed to absorb impact, while a firmer base layer provides essential stability and support. This design aims to distribute plantar pressures evenly across the foot, helping to relieve high-pressure zones and prevent skin degradation, which can lead to complications, especially in individuals with diabetes or other neurological conditions. On the other hand, rigid orthoses are made primarily from materials such as thermoplastics and carbon fiber. While they offer superior longevity and exceptional support, their rigid structure poses a challenge when fitting them to the unique contours of the foot [25]. These orthoses are often difficult to modify or reshape, which can limit their applicability for different foot shapes and conditions. Their main advantage lies in providing outstanding control and support, making them suitable for specific conditions requiring firm stabilization. Overall, selecting the right type of foot orthosis, whether accommodating, semirigid, or rigid, depends on the individual's specific needs, foot type, and the nature of their activities, ensuring optimal health and comfort.

6.4 Conventional Techniques for Orthosis Fabrication

In the conventional methodology of foot orthoses fabrication, the process begins with obtaining an imprint of the patient's foot. This imprint is crucial as it serves as the foundation for creating a custom-fit orthosis. Several techniques can be employed to capture this foot imprint, with options including 3D scanning, foam box impression, circumferential casting, and slipper casting. Each method has its own advantages and limitations, but they all aim to achieve an accurate representation of the foot's contours. Once the imprint is taken, a positive plaster cast is created from the negative mold of the foot. This involves pouring plaster into the obtained foot imprint, which hardens and forms a three-dimensional model of the patient's foot. Following this, a preheated thermoplastic sheet is placed over the positive plaster model, allowing it to conform to the precise shape of the foot [27]. While the basic manufacturing process can be accomplished using standard tools like measuring tapes and vernier calipers, obtaining precise, accurate measurements is essential for the effectiveness of the orthosis [28]. Depending on the materials used, accommodative foot orthoses can be physically molded to the patient's foot. This molding process can take advantage of the patient's body weight and heat, allowing the orthosis to adapt more closely to the individual's foot shape. Alternatively, external pressure and heat can be applied during the molding process to achieve a similar level of customization. Additionally, more advanced techniques such as Computer-Aided Design and Manufacturing (CAD-CAM) can be utilized to generate a negative imprint of the foot digitally. This digital footprint can enhance precision and streamline the process of creating the positive mold [25]. The positive mold is then utilized to vacuum form various materials, including carbon fiber and specialized plastic sheets, which are selected based on their performance and suitability for the intended use of the orthosis. After the vacuum molding process, the orthosis undergoes a meticulous finish, which may involve smoothing edges, applying cushioning materials, and ensuring that it meets the comfort and functional requirements before being delivered to the patient [29].

However, it is important to note that conventional manufacturing techniques often come with significant resource demands. They require specialized infrastructure conducive to the different stages of fabrication, such as dedicated areas for casting, modifying, finishing, and trial fittings. Additionally, a storage space for consumables like plaster powder and rolls is necessary [30]. The choice of design, the labor-intensive nature of the production process, and the extensive infrastructure requirements often present challenges in the conventional fabrication of orthoses. These factors can ultimately drive up both the cost and the duration of the fabrication process [31].

6.5 Diabetic Prevention Using Orthoses

The primary aim of diabetic care is to prevent the development or progression of foot ulcers, which can lead to serious complications if not managed effectively. Both surgical and nonsurgical approaches are utilized in this regard, allowing for a comprehensive treatment strategy tailored to the individual needs of the patient. Nonsurgical treatments play a crucial role, with methods such as the casting technique, particularly the total contact cast, being highly effective. This method helps to distribute pressure evenly across the foot, facilitating healing and reducing the risk of ulceration. Additionally, alterations in footwear are essential; options such as specially designed shoes, insoles, and in-shoe orthoses can provide necessary support and cushioning to alleviate pressure points [4]. Wearing appropriate socks can also contribute to comfort and moisture management, further mitigating ulcer risk. In addition to these measures, a variety of assistive devices can enhance patient mobility while ensuring foot protection. The use of walkers, braces, or canes can help to offload weight from the affected foot, allowing for safer ambulation. Other strategies include the use of felt padding to protect sensitive areas, plugs to fill voids in shoes, and wheelchairs for more long-term mobility support. Overall, a multifaceted approach, carefully balancing these nonsurgical interventions, is vital for effective diabetic foot care and preventing potentially serious complications such as ulcers.

Total contact casting is widely recognized as one of the most effective therapeutic approaches for managing DFUs. This method is particularly beneficial once an ulcer has completely healed, providing a supportive environment that promotes healing and protects the foot from further complications [25]. However, effective management of diabetic foot problems also necessitates preventative measures, primarily through the careful selection of orthotics and appropriate footwear. One of the key contributors to the development of foot ulcers in individuals with diabetes is the wearing of improperly fitted shoes. Shoes that do not conform well to the shape of the foot can lead to pressure points, friction, and ultimately ulceration. In contrast, well-fitting footwear serves a dual purpose: it significantly reduces the risk of foot ulceration while enhancing comfort by providing stability and support to existing foot deformities [32, 33]. The design and fit of shoes play a crucial role in distributing weight evenly across the foot and alleviating pressure from vulnerable areas. In managing diabetic foot health, several goals must be pursued through effective footwear management. These include protecting the foot from injury, relieving pressure on affected areas, reducing stress and shear forces, and accommodating the use of foot orthoses [34, 35].

To achieve these goals, healthcare providers must consider various factors when recommending footwear, including the patient's level of physical activity, unique foot shape, and overall skin health. For individuals who have never experienced ulcers, a well-fitting pair of commercially available shoes may suffice. However, those with a history of foot ulcers often require specialized footwear, which may involve a more complex prescription tailored to their specific needs. This bespoke approach ensures that the shoes provide the necessary features to protect the feet and promote healing. Diabetic foot orthoses, which are custom-made inserts, also play a vital role in maintaining foot health [32]. They offer shock absorption, promote even distribution of plantar pressure, shield sensitive areas from impact, reduce shear forces, and accommodate both flexible and fixed foot deformities. By addressing these needs, foot orthoses can significantly enhance the quality of life for individuals living with diabetes, further reducing the risk of complications associated with diabetic foot conditions.

Despite the availability of standard orthotic devices, numerous challenges persist in effectively managing foot health, particularly for individuals prone to callus formation and ulcers. These orthotic devices often fall short of addressing the underlying conditions that contribute to increased foot pressure, which is a primary factor in ulcer development [36]. Research into the management of post-ulcer conditions is ongoing, with a strong emphasis on off-loading strategies as the cornerstone of treatment. Off-loading involves redistributing weight away from ulcerated areas to promote healing and prevent further complications. Common options for off-loading include various modalities such as partial shoes that limit weight-bearing on affected foot regions, crutches that assist mobility while alleviating stress on the foot, wheelchairs that provide an alternative means of transport, and custom-made splints that offer targeted support. Additionally, therapeutic footwear designed with specialized insoles can help manage pressure distribution, while removable cast walkers provide protection and stability during the healing process. Ankle–foot orthoses (AFOs) are particularly beneficial as they not only relieve pressure from the plantar surface but also enable necessary movement at the ankle joint (see Fig. 6.2). This dual approach enhances a patient's ability to walk and engage in daily activities, ultimately improving their

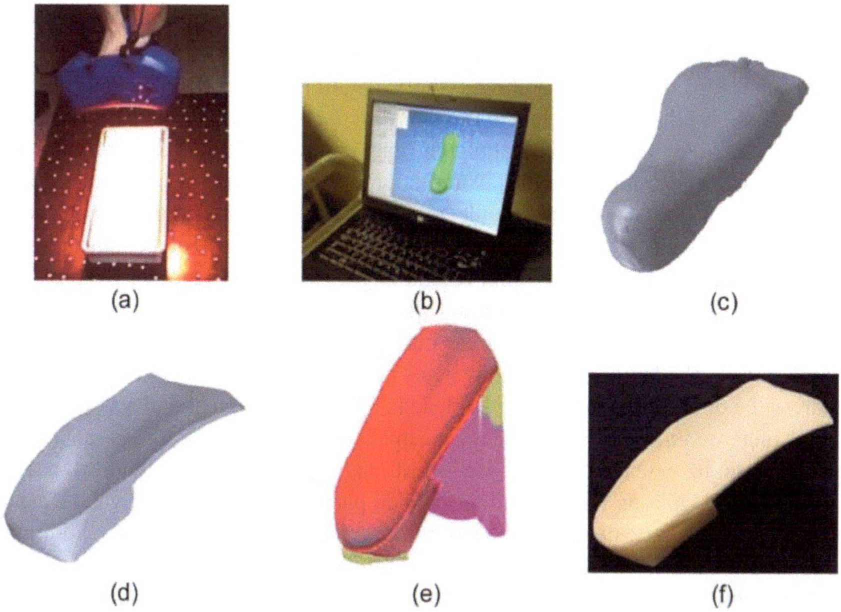

Fig. 6.2 Procedure of additive manufacturing for orthosis: **a** 3D scanning of the foam box, **b** Geometry modification, **c** Modified STL file of a positive foot model, **d** Merged FO (insole and heel), **e** FO setup for AM, and **f** FO made by FDM. *Reproduced under the terms of the Creative Commons Attribution 4.0 International License* [32]

overall mobility and quality of life. To ensure effective management of post-ulcer conditions, it is essential to employ a comprehensive approach that integrates these diverse treatment strategies [37]. This tailored care must take into account the individual patient's needs, the specific underlying conditions contributing to their foot problems, and the necessity for ongoing assessment and adjustment of the treatment plan. By prioritizing the implementation of these multifaceted strategies, healthcare providers can significantly improve patient outcomes and reduce the risk of recurrence [38].

6.6 Management of Post-Ulcer Diabetic Foot Using Orthoses

Numerous clinical studies emphasize that individuals suffering from post-ulcer foot disease require effective off-loading to promote optimal healing. The use of functional orthoses plays a critical role in this process. These orthoses can be categorized into three main types: semiflexible, stiff, and flexible. Semiflexible orthoses feature strong rubber posts and arch support, providing a balance of stability and mobility. Stiff orthoses, made from heat-moldable plastic materials, offer a rigid structure that helps manage foot pressure effectively. Lastly, flexible orthoses, composed of materials such as felt, rubber, and foam, provide cushioning and adapt to various foot shapes [39]. In addition to these orthotic solutions, conventional treatments for calluses involve the regular application of moisturizers, the careful paring of hyperkeratotic skin, and the use of hypoallergenic cushioning to alleviate discomfort. Total contact casting has long been a favored approach for treating ulcers, particularly in the early stages of neuropathic ulcers. This method is advantageous because it redistributes weight and reduces pressure on the affected areas. Total contact casting encompasses the entire lower limb, resembling a sock, and is crafted from plaster with minimal padding. This design allows for even distribution of vertical forces while effectively reducing shear stress during ambulation. Despite the benefits of standard orthotic devices, many challenges persist [40]. These devices often fail to address the underlying conditions that lead to callus formation and ulcers, primarily due to increased foot pressure. The management of post-ulcer conditions remains an area of ongoing research, and off-loading strategies continue to be the most essential approach. Options for off-loading include partial shoes, crutches, wheelchairs, custom-made splints, therapeutic footwear, and removable cast walkers. Additionally, AFOs designed to relieve pressure can significantly aid in unloading the plantar surface, while also facilitating movement at the ankle joint, ultimately enhancing the patient's mobility and quality of life [41]. Understanding and implementing these diverse treatment strategies is crucial for effective management of post-ulcer conditions, ensuring that patients receive comprehensive care tailored to their specific needs.

6.7 Customized Insoles

Insoles have emerged as a crucial intervention in the prevention and management of DFUs, a serious complication that affects many individuals with diabetes. These ulcers are often caused by increased pressure and poor circulation, making the selection of appropriate insoles important. Research underscores that custom-contoured insoles significantly outperform standard flat insoles, often made from pressure-relieving materials, when it comes to alleviating plantar surface pressure. Notably, studies by Cheung and Zhang, Goske et al., and Luo et al. [42–44] indicate that these customized designs are particularly beneficial for patients already suffering from DFUs or those at high risk of developing them. The incorporation of arch support in insole designs plays a critical role in enhancing both comfort and efficacy. By strategically redistributing plantar stresses, these insoles protect vulnerable areas beneath the metatarsal heads, which are often prone to ulceration. Cheung and Zhang [43] emphasize that this targeted support not only alleviates discomfort but also promotes even weight distribution during ambulation, reducing the likelihood of pressure build-up. Innovative developments in insole design have introduced models like the one proposed by Dai et al. [45], featuring a distinct layer designed to mimic the properties of a sock. Their experimental findings revealed that wearing socks while walking could result in a remarkable reduction, over 80%, in plantar shear stresses compared to walking barefoot. This significant reduction in shear stress is critically important for individuals with diabetes, as lower shear forces can drastically mitigate the risk of ulcer formation.

The ongoing use of insoles is widely regarded as a foundational treatment strategy for individuals grappling with DFUs. In recent years, advancements in finite element modeling (FEM) have enabled researchers to conduct in-depth investigations into the efficacy of various insole designs in mitigating plantar pressure and facilitating recovery from foot ulcers. For instance, Lemmon et al. [46] employed a two-dimensional FE model that simulated the sagittal adjustment of the second metatarsal along with key anatomical elements, including soft tissue, insole design, and midsole characteristics. Their research uncovered that custom-designed insoles could lead to a reduction in plantar pressure by as much as 29%. This significant alleviation of pressure is imperative for the healing process, as it offloads stress from affected areas, thereby fostering recovery. Luo et al. [44] conducted an in-depth study utilizing a two-dimensional (2D) foot model that incorporated essential anatomical components, including the calcaneus bone, heel pad, skin, and insoles with varying degrees of stiffness. This model was specifically analyzed to understand the conditions to assess how different insoles impacted diabetic patients' foot health. The study systematically compared the biomechanical responses produced by custom-designed insoles against traditional barefoot conditions. The findings revealed that the use of custom-based insoles significantly alleviated stress and strain energy density in the feet, showing a marked reduction in internal stresses at the plantar fascia, compared to those near the calcaneus bone. This differential stress distribution indicates that custom insoles not only better support the foot's structure but also effectively target areas that are most vulnerable to injury in diabetic patients. Furthermore, the study underscored the importance of finite element modeling in the research process, providing valuable insights into the effectiveness of various insole types in mitigating plantar pressure, a critical factor in managing diabetic foot conditions. The data suggested that the tailored design of custom insoles results in superior performance, effectively reducing plantar pressure more than flat insoles, which typically do not conform to the individual needs of patients [4, 32, 47]. Overall, the development and implementation of custom-made insoles (CMIs) represent a significant advancement in therapeutic strategies for improving foot health in individuals with diabetes, as illustrated in Fig. 6.3, which details the step-by-step process of creating these specialized insoles for diabetic patients.

Numerous comprehensive research studies have been conducted to investigate the benefits of incorporating pressure-relieving plugs into insoles or footwear specifically designed for diabetic patients suffering from foot ulcers. These studies have primarily focused on critical anatomical areas, particularly the forefoot and heel, which are most vulnerable to pressure-related injuries that can exacerbate ulceration and lead to complications. One significant study by Erdemir et al. [49] examined the effects of pressure-relieving plugs on the peak pressures endured by the foot during typical activities. Their findings indicated a substantial reduction in peak pressures experienced under the metatarsal head when these plugs were employed.

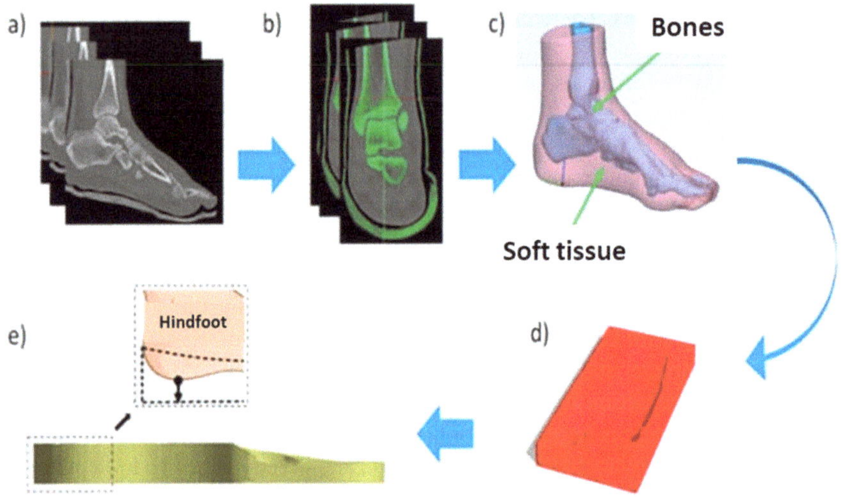

Fig. 6.3 Finite element model generation through various steps including: **a** The computerized tomography (CT) scan images of foot, **b** Processed CT images with segmentation, **c** Reconstructed foot model with bones and soft tissue, **d** Subtracted foot from box to construct a CMI, and **e** CMI dimensions following the foot morphology and length. *Reproduced under the terms of the Creative Commons Attribution 4.0 International License* [48]

The researchers conducted simulation experiments that emphasized the importance of strategic placement of the plugs; they found that positioning the plug at the apex of the pressure distribution yielded more pronounced results than merely placing it directly beneath the metatarsal head. This highlights the necessity of considering not only the use of pressure-relieving devices but also their precise positioning to maximize therapeutic effects and optimize foot protection. In a subsequent study, Actis et al. [50] explored the effects of smaller plugs, approximately 4 mm in size, utilizing a two-dimensional model of the whole foot with a focus on the cross-section of the second ray. Their objective was to examine how these smaller plugs could be integrated into total contact insoles under the metatarsal head. The results revealed that the incorporation of these diminutive plugs led to a measurable decrease in peak plantar pressures, indicating that even smaller interventions can be effective in alleviating pressure distribution across the foot. Further research by Gu et al. [51] shifted focus to the heel area, which is another critical zone for DFUs. This study concluded that the most efficient method to reduce plantar pressures involved utilizing a plug that was at least 10 mm in thickness made from medium hardness material, with a diameter that corresponded to 95% of the calcaneus. This attention to the specific dimensions and material properties of the plugs is crucial for ensuring optimal pressure relief and highlights the significance of tailored solutions for individual patient needs.

In a significant contribution to the field of diabetic foot care, researchers led by Barani et al. [52] conducted a comprehensive study examining the efficacy of silicone gel insoles in alleviating pressure on diabetic foot. Their research utilized advanced three-dimensional stress analysis techniques to assess diabetic insoles, focusing on various loading points across the surface of the foot. The findings underscored that the precise alignment of the insole with the unique shape of the foot was a critical factor in reducing pressure on the plantar surface. This research highlighted the essential need for customized insole designs that are specifically tailored to the individual anatomies of patients, thereby improving comfort and potentially preventing complications associated with diabetic foot conditions. Similarly, another pivotal study conducted by Goske et al. [42] explored a two-dimensional model of the heel region, which included the calcaneus, surrounding soft tissues, and the insole. This study aimed to investigate the impact of different variables, such as insole thickness, material composition, and degree of conformity, specifically for diabetic patients. The results reaffirmed the earlier findings, indicating that the degree of conformity of the insole to the foot's contours was a significant determinant in reducing pressure on the plantar surface. Further advancing the field, Budhabhatti et al. [53] developed a detailed foot model and examined various insole materials under specific foot conditions commonly experienced during push-off and toe-off phases of walking. Their rigorous assessments revealed that different insole materials could lead to a substantial reduction in peak plantar pressure. Specifically, they found that the use of specialized insole materials decreased peak pressures at the first metatarsal head by 18–69% and at the hallux by 49–68%, compared to the barefoot condition. These findings not only illustrate the potential of tailored insole materials to enhance mobility and comfort for diabetic patients but also pave the way for future research into personalized orthopedic solutions.

In summary, the advancement and use of custom insoles mark a significant improvement in diabetic foot care. These specially designed insoles have been shown to be more effective at reducing plantar pressure compared to traditional flat insoles, ultimately leading to better health outcomes for individuals at risk of diabetic foot complications. Continued innovation and research hold great promise for enhancing the quality of life for those affected by diabetes. However, there is still a lack of effective, patient-specific pressure offloading devices tailored to address the risk of ulcers at various locations on the foot. Developing such customized offloading solutions is crucial for preventing ulcers by ensuring that pressure distribution is optimized according to each individual's unique anatomical and physiological needs. Through these advancements, we can improve care for those at risk of diabetic foot complications.

References

1. Owings TM et al (2009) Plantar pressures in diabetic patients with foot ulcers which have remained healed. Diabet Med 26:1141–1146
2. Singh G, Chanda A (2024) Finite element modeling of diabetic foot: a state-of-the-art review. Eng. Res. Express 6:012507

3. Singh G, Lamba A, Chanda A (2024) Role of additive manufacturing for the management of diabetic foot ulcers. In Addit Manuf Biomed Appl 19–38 (Springer, Singapore). https://doi.org/10.1007/978-981-97-5456-4_2
4. Singh G, Bose D, Chanda A (2025) Development and Testing of a Novel Diabetic Orthosis for Plantar Pressure Reduction. Facta Univ Ser Mech Eng. https://doi.org/10.22190/FUME240725044S
5. Oyibo SO et al (2001) The effects of ulcer size and site, patient's age, sex and type and duration of diabetes on the outcome of diabetic foot ulcers. Diabet Med 18:133–138
6. Singh G, Chanda A (2022) Biomechanical modeling of progressive wound healing: A computational study. Biomed Eng Adv. 4:100055
7. Pourghasem M, Kamali N, Farsi M, Soltanpour N (2016) Prevalence of flatfoot among school students and its relationship with BMI. Acta Orthop Traumatol Turc 50:554–557
8. Filardi V (2018) Flatfoot and normal foot a comparative analysis of the stress shielding. J Orthop 15:820–825
9. Niu J, Liu J, Zheng Y, Ran L, Chang Z (2020) Are arch-conforming insoles a good fit for diabetic foot? Insole customized design by using finite element analysis. Hum Factors Ergon Manuf Serv Ind. 30:303–310
10. Caputo GM, Cavanagh PR, Ulbrecht JS, Gibbons GW, Karchmer AW (1994) Assessment and management of foot disease in patients with diabetes. N Engl J Med 331:854–860
11. Turner DE, Helliwell PS, Burton AK, Woodburn J (2007) The relationship between passive range of motion and range of motion during gait and plantar pressure measurements. Diabet Med 24:1240–1246
12. Chanda A, Unnikrishnan V (2018) Novel insole design for diabetic foot ulcer management. Proc Inst Mech Eng Part H J Eng Med. 232, 1182–1195
13. Dubský M et al (2013) Risk factors for recurrence of diabetic foot ulcers: prospective follow-up analysis in the Eurodiale subgroup. Int Wound J 10:555–561
14. Dragoi II, Popescu FG, Bowling FL, Bondor CI, Ionac M (2023) Patients' buying behavior for non-reimbursed off-loading devices used in diabetic foot ulcer treatment—an observational study during COVID-19 pandemic from a romanian physical therapy unit. J Clin Med 12, Page 6516 12, 6516
15. Gupta V, Chanda A (2022) Biomechanics of skin grafts: effect of pattern size, spacing and orientation. Eng Res Express 4:015006
16. Singh G, Chanda A (2021) Mechanical properties of whole-body soft human tissues : a review. Biomed Mater 16:062004
17. Makode S, Singh G, Chanda A (2021) Development of novel anisotropic skin simulants. Phys Scr 96:125019
18. Singh G, Gupta V, Chanda A (2022) Artificial skin with varying biomechanical properties. Mater Today Proc. 62:3162–3166
19. Andersen H, Gjerstad MD, Jakobsen J (2004) Atrophy of Foot MusclesA measure of diabetic neuropathy. Diabetes Care 27:2382–2385
20. Driver VR, Fabbi M, Lavery LA, Gibbons G (2010) The costs of diabetic foot: The economic case for the limb salvage team. J Vasc Surg 52:17S-22S
21. Nemcová J, Hlinková E (2014) The efficacy of diabetic foot care education. J Clin Nurs 23:877–882
22. Lim JZM, Ng NSL, Thomas C (2017) Prevention and treatment of diabetic foot ulcers. J R Soc Med 110:104–109
23. Landorf KB, Keenan AM (2000) Efficacy of foot orthoses. What does the literature tell us? J Am Podiatr Med Assoc 90, 149–158
24. Suglo JN, Winkley K, Sturt J (2022) Prevention and management of diabetes-related foot ulcers through informal caregiver involvement: a systematic review. J Diabetes Res. 2022
25. Janisse D, Janisse E (2015) Pedorthic management of the diabetic foot. Prosthet Orthot Int 39:40–47
26. Schrank ES, Stanhope SJ (2011) Dimensional accuracy of ankle-foot orthoses constructed by rapid customization and manufacturing framework. J Rehabil Res Dev 48:31–42

27. Chen RK, Jin Y an, Wensman J, Shih A (2016) Additive manufacturing of custom orthoses and prostheses—A review. Addit Manuf 12, 77–89
28. Dombroski CE, Balsdon MER, Froats A (2014) The use of a low cost 3D scanning and printing tool in the manufacture of custom-made foot orthoses: A preliminary study. BMC Res Notes 7:1–4
29. Farhan M, Wang JZ, Bray P, Burns J, Cheng TL (2021) Comparison of 3D scanning versus traditional methods of capturing foot and ankle morphology for the fabrication of orthoses: a systematic review. J Foot Ankle Res. 14:1–11
30. Chevalier TL, Chockalingam N (2012) Effects of foot orthoses: How important is the practitioner? Gait Posture 35:383–388
31. Totah D, Kovalenko I, Saez M, Barton K (2017) Manufacturing choices for ankle-foot orthoses: a multi-objective optimization. Procedia CIRP 65:145–150
32. Chhikara K, Singh G, Gupta S, Chanda A (2022) Progress of additive manufacturing in fabrication of foot orthoses for diabetic patients: A review. Ann 3D Print. Med. 8, 100085
33. Aalaa M, Malazy OT, Sanjari M, Peimani M, Mohajeri-Tehrani MR (2012) Nurses' role in diabetic foot prevention and care; a review. J Diabetes Metab Disord 11:1–6
34. Gupta S, Singh G, Chanda A (2021) Prediction of diabetic foot ulcer progression: a computational study. Biomed Phys Eng Express 7:065020
35. Singh G, Gupta S, Chanda A (2021) Biomechanical modelling of diabetic foot ulcers: A computational study. J Biomech 127:110699
36. Brodsky JW, Kourosh S, Stills M, Mooney V (1988) Objective evaluation of insert material for diabetic and athletic footwear. Foot Ankle Int 9:111–116
37. Caselli A, Pham H, Giurini JM, Armstrong DG, Veves A (2002) The forefoot-to-rearfoot plantar pressure ratio is increased in severe diabetic neuropathy and can predict foot ulceration. Diabetes Care 25:1066–1071
38. Boulton AJM et al (1984) Reduction of abnormal foot pressures in diabetic neuropathy using a new polymer insole material. Diabetes Care 7:42–46
39. Colagiuri S, Marsden LL, Naidu V, Taylor L (1995) The use of orthotic devices to correct plantar callus in people with diabetes. Diabetes Res Clin Pract 28:29–34
40. Ali A et al (2017) Fibreglass Total Contact Casting, Removable Cast Walkers, and Irremovable Cast Walkers to Treat Diabetic Neuropathic Foot Ulcers: A Health Technology Assessment. Ont. Health Technol. Assess. Ser. 17:1
41. Chakraborty PP et al (2015) A comparative study between total contact cast and pressure-relieving ankle foot orthosis in diabetic neuropathic foot ulcers. J Diabetes Sci Technol 9:302–308
42. Goske S, Erdemir A, Petre M, Budhabhatti S, Cavanagh PR (2006) Reduction of plantar heel pressures: Insole design using finite element analysis. J Biomech 39:2363–2370
43. Cheung JTM, Zhang M (2005) A 3-dimensional finite element model of the human foot and ankle for insole design. Arch Phys Med Rehabil 86:353–358
44. Luo G, Houston VL, Garbarini MA, Beattie AC, Thongpop C (2011) Finite element analysis of heel pad with insoles. J Biomech 44:1559–1565
45. Dai XQ, Li Y, Zhang M, Cheung JTM (2006) Effect of sock on biomechanical responses of foot during walking. Clin Biomech 21:314–321
46. Lemmon D, Shiang TY, Hashmi A, Ulbrecht JS, Cavanagh PR (1997) The effect of insoles in therapeutic footwear—A finite element approach. J Biomech 30:615–620
47. Gupta S et al (2023) Diabot: development of a diabetic foot pressure tracking device. J 6, 32–47
48. Nouman M, Dissaneewate T, Chong DYR, Chatpun S (2021) Effects of Custom-Made Insole Materials on Frictional Stress and Contact Pressure in Diabetic Foot with Neuropathy: Results from a Finite Element Analysis. Appl Sci 11, Page 3412
49. Erdemir A et al (2005) Local plantar pressure relief in therapeutic footwear: design guidelines from finite element models. J Biomech 38:1798–1806
50. Actis RL et al (2008) Multi-plug insole design to reduce peak plantar pressure on the diabetic foot during walking. Med Biol Eng Comput 46:363–371

51. Gu Y, Li J, Ren X, Lake MJ, Zeng Y (2010) Heel skin stiffness effect on the hind foot biomechanics during heel strike. Ski. Res. Technol. 16:291–296
52. Barani Z, Haghpanahi M, Katoozian H (2005) Three dimensional stress analysis of diabetic insole: A finite element approach. Technol Heal Care 13:185–192
53. Budhabhatti SP et al (2007) Finite Element Modeling of the First Ray of the Foot: A Tool for the Design of Interventions. J Biomech Eng 129:750–756

Chapter 7
Development of Modular Insole and Pressure Measurement Device

7.1 Introduction

In recent years, significant advancements in the analysis of foot pressure have led to the creation of highly customized insoles designed to meet individual needs, thereby enhancing both ergonomics and comfort. These insoles play a critical role by providing cushioning precisely at the points where the foot makes contact with the inside of the footwear. The design and material selection for these insoles are not merely aesthetic choices; they have a profound influence on how plantar pressure is distributed across the foot [1, 2]. Understanding the biomechanics of foot movement and pressure distribution is essential for optimizing these designs. Researchers have employed advanced pressure mapping technology to gain insights into the various pressure points experienced during activities such as walking, running, and standing [3, 4]. By identifying high-pressure areas, they can develop insoles that effectively alleviate stress on the feet, reducing discomfort and the risk of injury. Moreover, the appropriate insoles not only enhance foot protection but also contribute significantly to overall wearing comfort. This increased comfort can lead to improved performance in daily activities, making even the most routine tasks feel more effortless. Ultimately, the combination of tailored design, proper material use, and cutting-edge technology results in insoles that support better foot health, enhance mobility, and promote a more comfortable experience throughout the day [5, 6].

When addressing the treatment of diabetic foot ulcers, it is important to recognize that these ulcers commonly develop due to repetitive or excessive mechanical pressure on areas of insensitive skin. This ongoing pressure can lead to significant tissue damage, impede the healing process, and even result in serious complications if not managed properly [7, 8]. Heel ulcers, in particular, pose unique challenges in treatment. A prevalent approach involves the use of custom-designed insoles that feature a hole or cushioning material strategically placed beneath the active wound site. These insoles are intended to reduce normal and shear stresses on the ulcerated area, providing relief and aiding the healing process [9, 10]. However, a critical

A. Chanda and G. Singh, *Diabetic Foot Ulcer*, Biomedical Materials for Multi-functional Applications, https://doi.org/10.1007/978-981-95-2484-6_7

concern arises regarding the interaction between mechanical loads and these insoles. The design of the insoles can create pressure focal points at the edges of the hole due to the abrupt transition in material properties. This sudden change can amplify external forces at the perimeter of the wound, counteracting the intended therapeutic benefits and increasing the risk of developing secondary ulcers in nearby areas of the foot [11]. Conventional interventions for managing diabetic ulcers often focus on pressure offloading techniques. These techniques may involve the use of crutches to completely remove weight-bearing from affected areas, specialized foot orthotics that are carefully tailored to redistribute pressure across the foot, and custom-designed pressure offloading insoles that deliver targeted alleviation to the ulcer site [12–14]. The primary goal of these medical interventions is to effectively redistribute the pressure exerted on the plantar fascia, a vital structure of the foot that supports normal walking and balance. When compromised, the plantar fascia can contribute to the formation of ulcers, making pressure redistribution crucial in preventing and treating these painful wounds. By addressing the mechanical aspects of foot ulcers comprehensively, it is possible to enhance healing outcomes and improve quality of life for individuals suffering from diabetes-related complications [15, 16].

7.2 Need for Customized Insoles

Customized foot insoles are increasingly recognized as a highly effective treatment option for individuals experiencing various foot-related issues. This effectiveness is largely due to their design, which provides complete contact with the plantar surface of the foot. By ensuring full surface area interaction, these insoles help distribute body weight more evenly, offering better support and stability compared to traditional prefabricated orthotics [16, 17]. Research has highlighted the critical role of these customized orthotics, especially for diabetic patients. Studies indicate that they can significantly reduce plantar pressures, thereby lowering the risk of developing diabetic foot ulcers, a common complication of diabetes that can lead to serious health consequences [18–20]. In particular, a study by Caselli et al. [21] revealed that areas such as the forefoot and heel are exceptionally susceptible to high plantar pressure levels in diabetic individuals. This excessive pressure not only leads to discomfort but also correlates positively with the severity of neuropathic diseases. As neuropathy advances, so does the risk of foot injuries, including painful and potentially debilitating ulcers. To further investigate the relationship between plantar pressure and gait dynamics, Cock et al. [22] utilized a sophisticated force-measuring device that allowed for precise assessment of both the center of pressure and the overall plantar pressure throughout various phases of walking. Their findings revealed significant variability in plantar pressure across different gait stages, suggesting that the forces exerted on the foot can change with each step taken. This variability underscores the need for tailored treatment approaches and careful monitoring, as it can greatly influence both diagnosis and subsequent therapeutic measures for individuals with foot-related complications. Through these insights, the importance of customized insoles becomes even clearer, as they can adapt to these changes and provide the necessary support to mitigate risks associated with high plantar pressures.

The development of sensor-based insoles marks a notable advancement in the realm of diabetic foot care, bringing innovative solutions directly into the lives of patients. These insoles are designed to collect detailed pressure data in real time, even outside of clinical environments, which facilitates ongoing monitoring and allows for the early identification of potential foot issues [23, 24]. This capability is particularly crucial for diabetic patients, who are at an elevated risk for foot complications due to impaired circulation and reduced sensation. Additionally, a variety of studies have investigated the efficacy of shoe-based pressure-measuring devices that operate during walking or running. Many of these advanced devices utilize cutting-edge technologies, such as force-sensitive resistors and piezoresistive materials. These technologies enhance the flexibility of the sensors, enabling them to provide more accurate and comfortable measurements of foot pressure during various activities [25]. This ongoing research highlights the critical role of technological integration in diabetic foot care, aiming to enhance patient outcomes and reduce the likelihood of severe complications, such as foot ulcers. A thorough review of existing literature reveals that custom pressure offloading insoles deliver benefits comparable to those of the total contact cast (TCC), yet with fewer associated drawbacks. These specialized insoles are crafted to redistribute pressure away from vulnerable areas of the foot, which is particularly important for diabetic patients who are susceptible to developing foot ulcers. The customization process, however, is labor-intensive and demands attention to detail. Each insole must be specifically designed to fit an individual's unique foot shape and pressure distribution patterns, significantly enhancing its effectiveness in preventing injuries [26, 27]. Unfortunately, traditional methods for fabricating these custom insoles can be time consuming, often requiring several days to produce a device that effectively isolates and alleviates pressure from ulcer-prone areas. As such, advancements in manufacturing processes and technology are necessary to streamline the creation of these vital assistive devices, ultimately leading to better patient care and prevention of foot-related complications [28–30].

To effectively address the challenges faced by individuals with diabetic foot conditions, there is a pressing need for the development of a tailored, cost-effective insole that can be adapted to suit a wide range of foot shapes and medical conditions. This innovative insole should not only target and alleviate pressure in specific high-risk areas of the diabetic foot but also provide exceptional comfort and shock absorption, particularly in the heel region, which is often subjected to significant impact during daily activities. Moreover, the design must ensure comprehensive support across the entire plantar surface. This is essential for maintaining proper foot function and preventing the development of ulcers, which can lead to serious complications. Our research focused on creating and validating a customized modular insole that is specifically designed to redistribute and off-load plantar pressure for diabetic patients, particularly in areas most susceptible to ulceration. This modular insole concept allows for adjustments and personalization based on the individual patient's foot anatomy and pressure distribution patterns. By doing so, it aims to effectively prevent ulceration not only during postoperative medical care but also throughout ongoing wound management. Through this innovative approach, we envision a significant improvement in the quality of life for diabetic patients, helping them to better manage their foot health and maintain mobility.

7.3 Modular Insole for Plantar Pressure Offloading

The modular diabetic pressure offloading insole is thoughtfully engineered to deliver targeted relief and support for individuals suffering from ulcerated areas on their foot, an all-too-common complication for people with diabetes. This innovative insole incorporates removable supporting segments designed to create a therapeutic void beneath the affected areas. By doing so, it promotes even weight distribution across the foot, significantly reducing pressure on ulcerated spots and paving the way for faster healing. Constructed from high-quality, durable materials, this insole does not sacrifice comfort for functionality. It is designed for everyday wear, providing the essential cushioning and support needed to keep feet comfortable and pain free. Advanced manufacturing techniques have been employed to ensure each component of the insole can adapt to a wide variety of foot shapes and sizes, while still maintaining stability and support throughout the walking cycle. In addition to enhancing comfort, the design prioritizes the needs of diabetic patients, who often face challenges related to foot health. By mitigating pressure points and facilitating better circulation, this novel insole not only aims to improve the quality of life for users but also serves as a potential game-changer in the management of diabetes and the treatment of foot ulcers. Its novel design is a significant step forward in preventative foot care, promoting overall well-being for individuals with diabetes.

7.3.1 Designing and Modeling of Modular Insole

A standard UK-8 insole size was chosen as the foundational reference for the design and fabrication of the modular insole system. To ensure precision in the development process, the outline of the insole's mid-frame was precisely plotted utilizing the Mondopoint sizing system through Solid Works 2021 (Dassault Systèmes, France). This advanced software facilitated precise dimensional adjustments tailored to accommodate varying foot morphologies, promoting optimal fit and comfort. The modular insole is comprised of two main components: the mid-frame, which is depicted in Fig. 7.1b, and fourteen uniquely molded silicone rubber inserts, illustrated in Fig. 7.1a. Each silicone insert was engineered to address specific anatomical zones of the foot, reflecting a user-centric design philosophy aimed at enhancing comfort and functionality. These molded inserts are designed to be both removable and reattachable, empowering users to personalize their insoles according to their unique comfort preferences and foot needs. This innovative segmentation strategy was informed by extensive research, which highlighted critical zones of the foot

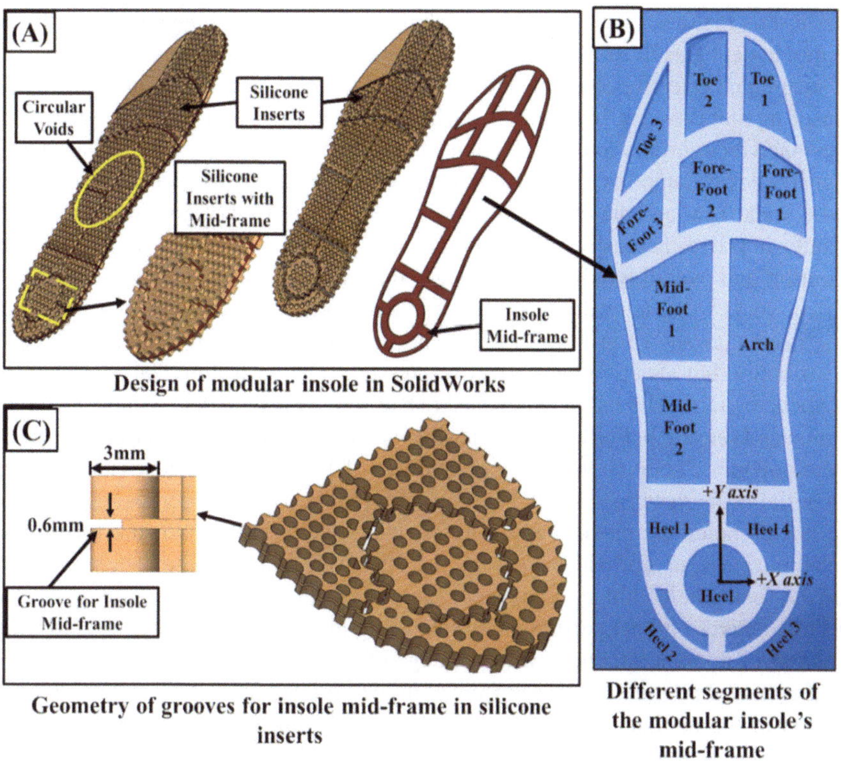

Fig. 7.1 **a** SolidWorks design of modular insole, **b** 3D-printed mid-frame for holding the inserts, and **c** Grooves geometry in inserts. *Reproduced with permission from the Publisher* [33]

that require targeted support. The study particularly focused on areas where diabetic patients frequently experience abnormal or elevated plantar pressures, underscoring the importance of delivering customized support solutions to mitigate potential complications associated with foot health. By allowing for this level of customization, the modular insole aims to foster improved foot care and overall well-being for its users [31, 32].

7.3.2 3D-Printing of Molds and Fabrication of Modular Insole

Given the significant stretching and bending strains experienced during walking, a thermoplastic polyurethane (TPU) material with a shore hardness of 95A was selected for the 3D printing of the mid-frame. This particular material, with a thickness of 0.6 mm, is engineered to withstand the dynamic stress conditions associated with daily activities, providing both durability and flexibility [34, 35]. The design of the inserts features specific grooves, each precisely measuring 0.6 mm in width and 3 mm in depth, as illustrated in Fig. 7.1c. These grooves are essential for facilitating a secure and effective attachment to the corresponding segments in the mid-frame, ensuring stability and integration. Each insert is crafted to a thickness of 6 mm, designed thoughtfully to enhance comfort and support for individuals. This comprehensive design supports a more natural gait, which is particularly beneficial for those who walk, run, and stand for extended periods. The primary goal was to significantly improve the cushioning properties of the insoles, a critical factor for user comfort and overall foot health. To realize this objective, strategically placed cylindrical voids were innovatively designed in a uniform pattern and incorporated into the inserts, as shown in Fig. 7.1a. This novel approach not only optimizes weight distribution but also promotes effective pressure relief, a feature that is crucial for diabetic patients who face a heightened risk of foot ulceration due to impaired circulation and sensation. Furthermore, the silicone inserts were produced from a specialized polymeric solution with a shore hardness of 10A (liquid silicone rubber). This material is characterized by its bio-inert and wear-resistant properties, rendering it an ideal choice for medical applications. It is easy to mold, allowing for precise customization, and provides a cushioning effect that adapts to the unique contours of the foot. The combination of these innovative design elements ensures that the inserts deliver optimal performance, enhancing the wearer's comfort and reducing the risk of injuries associated with prolonged foot stress.

Figure 7.2 provides a detailed view of the 3D-printed molds utilized in the fabrication of the modular insole, accompanied by the finished silicone inserts. These molds were designed with precision to ensure that the silicone inserts fit seamlessly within the overall structure of the insole. In addition, Fig. 7.3 showcases the intricately designed 3D-printed mid-frame of the insole, which plays a crucial role in providing structural support. This mid-frame was carefully engineered to allow for smooth assembly of the silicone inserts, resulting in a cohesive, modular insole that adapts to the unique shape of each foot. Once the modular insole was fully assembled, it was packaged in an innovative pouch specifically designed for participant trials. This pouch was made from a soft and stretchable material, which not only protects the insole but also conforms to the natural contours and movements of the foot. This feature greatly enhances comfort and fit during everyday use. This modular insole, developed with the specific needs of diabetic patients in mind, embodies cutting-edge technology aimed at improving overall user comfort. By effectively reducing the risk of ulceration, a common complication among diabetic individuals, this insole promotes better foot health and aids in maintaining mobility and quality of life.

7.4 Pressure Measurement Insole

A crucial element of the development process was the integration of an advanced wearable pressure measurement insole. This innovative insole is designed to provide a detailed analysis of pressure distribution across its surface, enabling a thorough

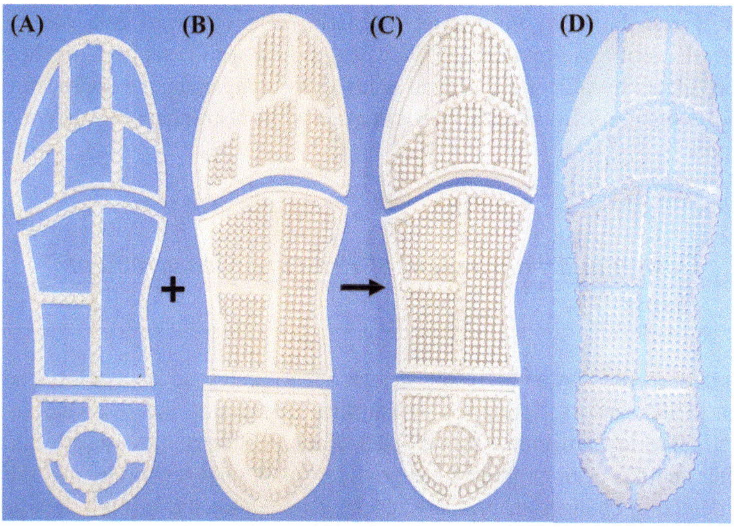

Fig. 7.2 **a** 3D-printed mold wall with grooves, **b** Mold base with circular voids, **c** Assembled mold for fabricating silicone inserts, **d** Fabricated silicone inserts. *Reproduced with permission from the Publisher* [33]

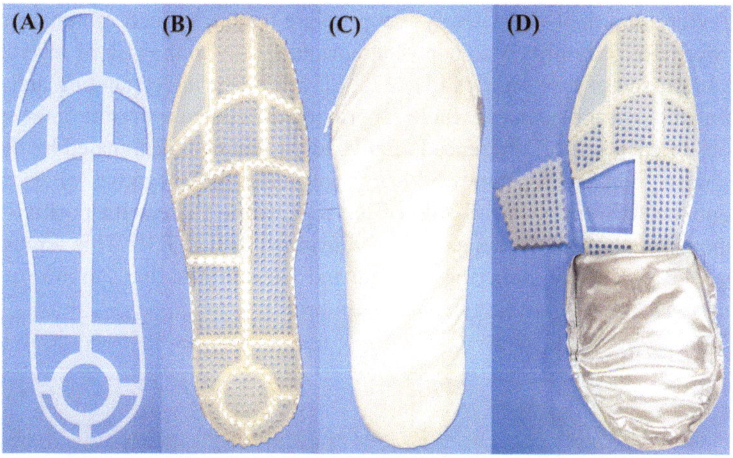

Fig. 7.3 **a** 3D printed mid-frame, **b** Assembled silicone inserts and mid-frame, **c** modular insole in the pouch, **d** Mid-foot 1 insert removed from the insole (for representation only). *Reproduced with permission from the Publisher* [33]

evaluation of its effectiveness in alleviating pressure from ulcerated areas. The system utilizes sensors to capture real-time data, which is then analyzed to identify high-pressure zones and monitor the insole's performance continuously. During the rigorous testing phase, various conditions were simulated to ensure the insole's reliability and durability in everyday scenarios. The collected data was carefully analyzed to verify its functionality, focusing on how well it supports the healing of pressure ulcers by offloading critical areas. This comprehensive approach ensures that the modular insole meets the needs of users while also enhancing patient comfort and safety.

7.4.1 Design and Fabrication of Pressure Measurement Insole

This pressure measurement insole design incorporates advanced force-sensitive resistor (FSR) sensors, developed by Interlink Electronics, Inc., a reputable manufacturer based in California, United States. Each FSR sensor measures 12.5 mm in diameter and has been engineered to provide exceptional sensitivity and reliability when detecting changes in pressure levels. To enhance the insole's functionality, the design includes a total of eleven strategically placed FSR sensors, which are distributed across various regions of the insole to ensure comprehensive data collection on pressure distribution, as illustrated in Fig. 7.4. However, it is important to note that three specific regions, namely Toe 3, Heel 2, and Heel 3, were excluded from the data collection process. This decision was made based on the small size of these regions and their consistently low-pressure readings. Such minimal pressure levels were deemed unlikely to contribute meaningfully to the risk of ulceration or the reoccurrence of foot injuries [31, 32, 36]. For better understanding and clarity regarding the sensor placement, Table 7.1 provides a detailed overview of the specific locations of each sensor, referenced relative to the segment designated by the Heel as the origin point. In this framework, any coordinates with negative values indicate positions located on the lateral side of the foot, while those with positive values correspond to the medial side, as further illustrated in Fig. 7.1b. This arrangement of sensors is crucial for gathering accurate and relevant data that can inform future interventions and improve foot health outcomes.

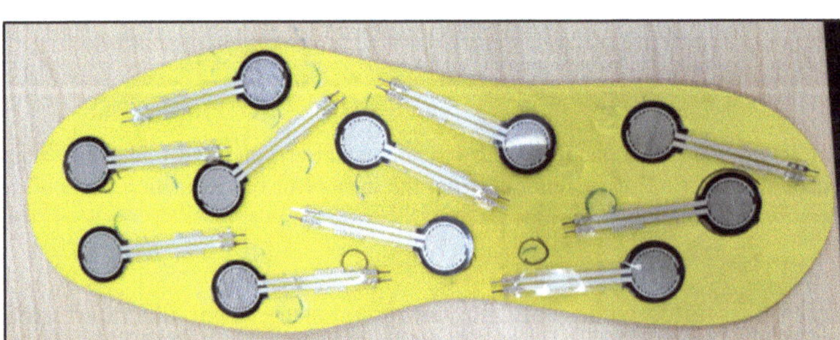

Fig. 7.4 FSR sensors at 11 different locations in the pressure-measuring insole. *Reproduced under the terms of the Creative Commons Attribution 4.0 International License* [37]

Table 7.1 Sensor location on the in-house fabricated pressure-measuring insole. *Reproduced with permission from the Publisher* [33]

Sensor location		Coordinates (in mm)	
Abbreviated word	Abbreviation	X-axis	Y-axis
Heel	Heel	0	0
Heel 4	Heel medial region	22.5	21
Heel 1	Heel lateral region	-22.5	21
Arch	Arch	14.5	86
Mid-Foot 2	Midfoot region 2	– 19	58
Mid-Foot 1	Midfoot region 1	– 22	110
Fore-Foot 3	Forefoot region 3	– 37	143
Fore-Foot 2	Forefoot region 2	– 6	161
Fore-Foot 1	Forefoot region 1	25	158
Toe 2	Toe region 2	– 9	207
Toe 1	Toe region 1 (Hallux)	16.5	203

Figure 7.5 presents a detailed illustration of the innovative pressure-measuring insole, precisely designed to capture the dynamic plantar pressure exerted by the foot during movement. The insole features an array of FSR sensors that were carefully affixed to one side of a 2 mm thick ethylene–vinyl acetate (EVA) foam sheet, which was custom-shaped to conform to the dimensions of a UK size 8 insole. This foundational layer not only enhances comfort but also ensures optimal contact with the foot, allowing the sensors to respond accurately to even subtle changes in pressure. To protect the sensors from potential damage and enhance the accuracy of the data collected, a 0.6 mm thick polylactic acid (PLA) sheet, produced through 3D printing technology, was attached to the opposite side of the EVA foam. This durable cover serves a dual purpose: it safeguards the sensitive FSR sensors from external impacts and deformation while providing a stable and consistent surface upon which pressure data can be reliably recorded during use. Each FSR sensor is integrated into a broader electrical system that includes a voltage divider circuit. This circuit plays a crucial role in regulating the output voltage from the sensors, ensuring that it is compatible with the input range of the microcontroller, which processes the data for analysis [38, 39]. The careful calibration of this system contributes significantly to the accuracy and reliability of the measurements obtained. For seamless data acquisition during experimental trials, a custom-designed 3D-printed enclosure was created to securely house the microcontroller board. This board was strategically positioned on the volunteer's leg with the aid of a Velcro strap, allowing it to remain stable and unmoving throughout the duration of data collection. A 20-band flat ribbon cable was utilized to connect the microcontroller to the embedded sensors within the insole, facilitating efficient and uninterrupted data transmission. By ensuring that the microcontroller board is firmly anchored in place, we significantly improve the integrity of the data collected, which enables a thorough and precise analysis of plantar pressure

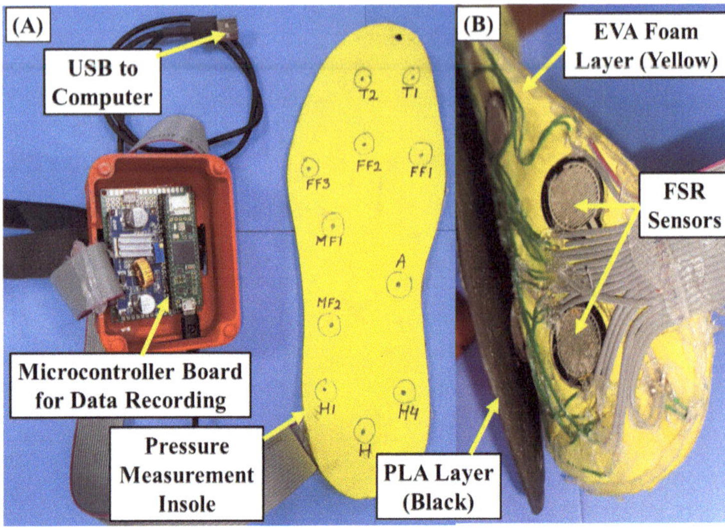

Fig. 7.5 **a** Pressure measuring insole with microcontroller board for data recording, and **b** EVA-PLA sandwich with FSR sensors. *Reproduced with permission from the Publisher* [33]

patterns throughout the study, ultimately contributing to a deeper understanding of foot dynamics.

7.5 Integration of Pressure Measurement Insole and Modular Offloading System

During the data collection phase of the study, the pressure-measuring insole was positioned beneath the modular insole within the shoe. This strategic placement was essential to ensure that the readings obtained were both accurate and reliable while also maintaining optimal comfort for the participant. To facilitate the collection and processing of pressure data, we employed the Arduino integrated development environment (IDE) to program the pressure-measuring insoles effectively. These advanced insoles were engineered to perform comprehensive scans at an exceptional rate of 5,000 scans per second. This high scanning frequency allowed for a nuanced and high-resolution analysis of plantar pressure, which is vital for understanding foot dynamics during various activities. A complete scan is defined as the duration it takes for the microcontroller to execute one full cycle of the programmed code. This process culminates in the display of processed values derived from each individual sensor embedded in the insole, providing a granular view of pressure distribution. To further enhance the depth of our analysis, we recorded the mean values of the plantar pressures at intervals of 20 ms for each scan. This rapid and high-resolution sampling frequency enabled us to capture dynamic changes in pressure distribution over time, offering valuable insights into how foot pressures fluctuate during movement. Overall, this careful and methodical approach to data collection allowed us to gather a rich dataset that significantly contributes to our understanding of plantar pressure dynamics.

The study not only examined mean pressure values but also tracked the maximum pressure readings recorded by each sensor throughout the entirety of the trial period. This dual focus on both average and peak pressures provided critical insights into specific areas of the foot that experienced the highest pressure, which is essential for understanding and analyzing the potential risk factors associated with foot ulceration. Throughout the trials, the extensive data collected were visually represented on a laptop using the Arduino IDE, as illustrated in Fig. 8.1. The graphical representation allowed for easier interpretation of the data and facilitated real-time analysis. After completing each trial, we ensured the complete datasets, which comprised all pertinent sensor measurements, were securely transferred from the microcontroller board to the laptop. This transfer was accomplished via a USB connection, guaranteeing that all information was accurately captured and prepared for subsequent in-depth analysis. This systematic approach to data handling not only preserved the integrity of the information but also streamlined the process of evaluating the relationship between pressure dynamics and the risk of foot ulcers.

References

1. Gupta S et al (2023) Diabot: development of a diabetic foot pressure tracking device. J 6, 32–47
2. Chhikara K, Singh G, Gupta S, Chanda A (2022) Progress of additive manufacturing in fabrication of foot orthoses for diabetic patients: A review. Ann 3D Print Med. 8, 100085
3. Farhat G et al (2024) Efficacy of customized insoles in the distribution of the diabetic foot pressure: A randomized and controlled clinical trial. J Bodyw Mov Ther 40:842–851
4. Jonnala UK, Sankineni R, Ravi Kumar Y (2023) Design and development of fused deposition modeling (FDM) 3D-Printed Orthotic Insole by using gyroid structure. J Mech Behav Biomed Mater 145, 106005
5. Singh G, Lamba A, Chanda A (2024) Role of additive manufacturing for the management of diabetic foot ulcers. In Addit Manuf Biomed Appl 19–38 (Springer, Singapore). https://doi.org/10.1007/978-981-97-5456-4_2
6. Malki A, Hajibozorgi M, Verkerke GJ, Dekker R, Hijmans JM (2024) Plantar pressure reduction in the heel region through self-adjusting insoles with a heel cup in standard and individualized rocker shoes. Clin Biomech 116:106281
7. Singh G, Chanda A (2022) Biomechanical modeling of progressive wound healing: A computational study. Biomed Eng Adv. 4:100055
8. Scarton A et al (2018) A methodological framework for detecting ulcers' risk in diabetic foot subjects by combining gait analysis, a new musculoskeletal foot model and a foot finite element model. Gait Posture 60:279–285
9. Erdemir A et al (2005) Local plantar pressure relief in therapeutic footwear: design guidelines from finite element models. J Biomech 38:1798–1806
10. Wu SC, Jensen JL, Weber AK, Robinson DE, Armstrong DG (2008) Use of pressure offloading devices in diabetic foot ulcers do we practice what we preach? Diabetes Care 31:2118–2119
11. Shaulian H, Gefen A, Solomonow-Avnon D, Wolf A (2021) Finite element-based method for determining an optimal offloading design for treating and preventing heel ulcers. Comput Biol Med 131:104261

12. Chantelau E, Haage P (1994) An audit of cushioned diabetic footwear: relation to patient compliance. Diabet Med 11:114–116
13. Saliba Thorne C, Gatt A, DeRaffaele C, Bazena A, Formosa C (2021) Digital foot health technology and diabetic foot monitoring: A systematic review. Diabetes Res Clin Pract 175:108783
14. Malki A, Baltasar Badaya M, Dekker R, Verkerke GJ, Hijmans JM (2024) Effects of individually optimized rocker midsoles and self-adjusting insoles on plantar pressure in persons with diabetes mellitus and loss of protective sensation. Diabetes Res Clin Pract 207:111077
15. Jeffcoate WJ, Harding KG (2003) Diabetic foot ulcers. Lancet 361:1545–1551
16. Chhikara K, Gupta S, Chanda A (2022) Development of a novel foot orthosis for plantar pain reduction. Mater Today Proc. 62:3532–3537
17. Singh G, Chanda A (2024) Finite element modeling of diabetic foot: a state-of-the-art review. Eng Res Express 6:012507
18. Dunn JE et al (2004) Prevalence of foot and ankle conditions in a multiethnic community sample of older adults. Am J Epidemiol 159:491–498
19. Garrow AP, Silman AJ, Macfarlane GJ (2004) The cheshire foot pain and disability survey: A population survey assessing prevalence and associations. Pain 110:378–384
20. Hendry GJ, Fenocchi L, Woodburn J, Steultjens M (2018) Foot pain and foot health in an educated population of adults: results from the glasgow caledonian university alumni foot health survey. J Foot Ankle Res. 11:1–15
21. Caselli A, Pham H, Giurini JM, Armstrong DG, Veves A (2002) The forefoot-to-rearfoot plantar pressure ratio is increased in severe diabetic neuropathy and can predict foot ulceration. Diabetes Care 25:1066–1071
22. De Cock A, Vanrenterghem J, Willems T, Witvrouw E, De Clercq D (2008) The trajectory of the centre of pressure during barefoot running as a potential measure for foot function. Gait Posture 27:669–675
23. Pappas IPI, Popovic MR, Keller T, Dietz V, Morari M (2001) A reliable gait phase detection system. IEEE Trans Neural Syst Rehabil Eng 9:113–125
24. Tee KS et al (2017) A portable insole pressure mapping system. TELKOMNIKA (Telecommunication Comput Electron Control). 15, 1493–1500
25. Tang L et al (2019) Functional gradient structural design of customized diabetic insoles. J Mech Behav Biomed Mater 94:279–287
26. Mandolini M, Brunzini A, Germani M (2017) A collaborative web-based platform for the prescription of Custom-Made Insoles. Adv Eng Informatics 33:360–373
27. Paton JS, Stenhouse EA, Bruce G, Zahra D, Jones RB (2012) A comparison of customised and prefabricated insoles to reduce risk factors for neuropathic diabetic foot ulceration: A participant-blinded randomised controlled trial. J Foot Ankle Res. 5:1–11
28. Ma Z et al (2019) Design and 3D printing of adjustable modulus porous structures for customized diabetic foot insoles. Int J Light Mater Manuf. 2:57–63
29. Anderson J, Williams AE, Nester C (2020) Development and evaluation of a dual density insole for people standing for long periods of time at work. J Foot Ankle Res. 13:1–13
30. Ledoux WR et al (2013) Diabetic foot ulcer incidence in relation to plantar pressure magnitude and measurement location. J Diabetes Complications 27:621–626
31. Singh G, Gupta S, Chanda A (2021) Biomechanical modelling of diabetic foot ulcers: A computational study. J Biomech 127:110699
32. Gupta S, Singh G, Chanda A (2021) Prediction of diabetic foot ulcer progression: a computational study. Biomed Phys Eng Express 7:065020
33. Singh G, Bose D, Chanda A (2025) Development and testing of a novel diabetic orthosis for plantar pressure reduction. Facta Univ Ser Mech Eng. https://doi.org/10.22190/FUME240725044S
34. Singh G, Gupta V, Chanda A (2022) Mechanical characterization of rotating triangle shaped auxetic skin graft simulants. Facta Univ Ser Mech Eng. 0, 1–16
35. Turudija R, Stojković M, Stojković JR, Aranđelović J, Marinković D (2024) Stiffness of anatomically shaped lattice scaffolds made by direct metal laser sintering of Ti-6Al-4V powder: a comparison of two different design variants. Met 14, Page 219 14, 219

36. Chanda A, Unnikrishnan V (2018) Novel insole design for diabetic foot ulcer management. Proc Inst Mech Eng Part H J Eng Med 232, 1182–1195
37. Bose D, Singh G, Gupta S, Chanda A (2024) Development of a novel customized insole for effective pressure offloading in diabetic patients. Prosthesis 6:341–356
38. Li N, Yang D, Jiang L, Liu H, Cai H (2012) Combined Use of FSR sensor array and SVM classifier for finger motion recognition based on pressure distribution map. J Bionic Eng 9:39–47
39. Manna SK, Hannan Bin Azhar MA, Greace A (2023) Optimal locations and computational frameworks of FSR and IMU sensors for measuring gait abnormalities. Heliyon 9, e15210

Chapter 8
Clinical Study to Understand the Effectiveness of Plantar Pressure Offloading in Diabetic Patients

8.1 Introduction

This study presents a detailed clinical investigation aimed at evaluating the effectiveness of the novel modular insole specifically designed for offloading plantar pressure. The research involved two distinct groups of participants: one group comprised 15 healthy individuals, while the other consisted of 15 diabetic individuals. The primary goal was to ascertain the degree to which the modular insole could alleviate plantar pressure during both static standing and dynamic walking activities. To thoroughly assess the insole's performance, a series of in-shoe plantar pressure measurements was accurately conducted. These measurements utilized a custom-designed pressure-measuring insole that was equipped with force-sensitive resistors (FSR) sensors. This innovative setup allowed for highly accurate readings of plantar pressures across various conditions, capturing how the insole performed under different weights and activities. The results of this clinical study are expected to substantiate the hypothesis that the developed modular insole is effective in significantly reducing plantar pressure exerted on the foot. Such a reduction is particularly critical for diabetic individuals, as it could enhance overall comfort and play a vital role in the prevention of foot ulceration, a common and serious complication associated with diabetes [1, 2]. This research not only aims to validate the insole's design but also strives to contribute to better foot care solutions for vulnerable populations.

8.2 Performance of Modular Insole

The modular insole underwent a comprehensive evaluation involving both quantitative and qualitative methodologies, featuring a cohort of 30 male participants divided into two distinct groups: 15 healthy individuals and 15 males diagnosed with diabetes. All participants shared a common foot size of UK 8, ensuring uniformity in the study's

A. Chanda and G. Singh, *Diabetic Foot Ulcer*, Biomedical Materials for Multi-functional Applications, https://doi.org/10.1007/978-981-95-2484-6_8

findings. These trials were conducted in accordance with ethical standards approved by the Ethical Committee of the Indian Institute of Technology Delhi (IIT-Delhi), India. Detailed demographic information, as summarized in Table 8.1, was collected for each participant, encompassing vital attributes such as height, weight, and age. For the diabetic participants, additional health metrics, specifically blood glucose levels, were monitored and recorded. Notably, the glucose levels in the healthy participants ranged from 73 to 96 mg/dL, providing a baseline for comparison. The modular insole was tested rigorously across several performance parameters designed to assess its various functional aspects. These included user comfort, fit, durability, and pressure offloading capabilities. The objective was to ensure that the insole meets the highest safety and efficacy standards necessary for diabetic patients, who are particularly susceptible to foot complications. Each parameter was systematically evaluated to determine the insole's effectiveness in reducing the potential risks associated with foot issues in individuals with diabetes. Moreover, the study aimed to guarantee that the insole offers a comfortable and secure fit for all users, thereby enhancing their overall experience and well-being. Through these thorough evaluations, the research contributes valuable insights into the development of specialized footwear solutions tailored to the needs of both healthy individuals and those managing diabetes.

Table 8.1 Details of the healthy participants and those with diabetes for the study. *Reproduced with permission from the Publisher* [3]

Sr. no	Healthy participants			Participants with diabetes			
	Height (in cm)	Weight (in Kg)	Age (in years)	Height (in cm)	Weight (in Kg)	Age (in years)	Blood Glucose (mg/dL)
1	165.1	72	28	170.4	72	62	178.3
2	185.4	66	33	174.2	78	58	141.4
3	180.3	83	31	175.3	81	47	120.5
4	175.4	78	42	170.2	65	51	126.5
5	180.3	86	50	165.4	76	39	130.5
6	177.1	74	52	173.7	77	42	138.2
7	182.9	68	47	165.1	89	60	174.2
8	164.6	91	62	175.5	71	53	230.4
9	171.4	57	30	173.7	87	55	142.4
10	166.3	63	26	170.2	79	49	164.7
11	182.9	61	29	180.3	59	36	136.2
12	185.4	74	35	166.3	64	59	152.1
13	173.7	88	36	177.6	82	58	211.3
14	164.6	76	32	181.1	71	46	132.8
15	175.4	62	35	179.3	83	51	146.5

8.2.1 *Qualitative Tests*

The study was designed to comprehensively evaluate the performance of the modular insole using the Quebec User Evaluation of Satisfaction with Assistive Technology (QUEST 2.0) questionnaire [4, 5]. This detailed questionnaire is specifically geared towards measuring subjective user experiences with assistive devices, focusing on critical aspects such as comfort, ease of use, and overall effectiveness. It comprises eight items that participants rate on a scale from 1 to 5, where a score of 5 signifies complete satisfaction, and a score of 1 indicates complete dissatisfaction. To gain a deeper understanding of the insole's performance, the study involved two distinct groups: healthy participants (HP) and diabetic participants (DP). This division allowed for a more nuanced analysis of how different populations experience the product. The evaluation was conducted in two separate scenarios designed to assess the insoles under varying conditions. In the first scenario (Case 1 or Q1), the insole was tested with all inserts included in the mid-frame, providing an opportunity to assess its overall performance with maximum support and adaptability. In the second scenario (Case 2 or Q2), the study systematically removed the inserts one by one. This approach helped identify how the absence of each specific insert influenced user satisfaction and comfort levels, offering insights into which configurations were most effective for users. Overall, the study assessed four individual cases: healthy participants in Case 1 (HP-Q1) and Case 2 (HP-Q2), as well as diabetic participants in Case 1 (DP-Q1) and Case 2 (DP-Q2). By employing this structured approach, researchers could perform a detailed analysis of the modular insole's performance across different conditions and demographic groups. This comprehensive evaluation provided valuable insights into its efficacy, user satisfaction, and the specific needs of diverse user populations, helping to inform future design and development of assistive technologies.

8.2.2 *Quantitative Tests*

The testing setup consists of a pair of shoes, with one shoe outfitted with a pressure-measuring insole placed beneath a modular insole, effectively replacing its original insole (see Fig. 8.1). Trials were conducted under two distinct conditions: standing, referred to as case CS, and walking, referred to as case CW. Initially, each participant underwent comprehensive trials using the complete set of inserts integrated into the modular insole, which are documented as CS (full) for standing and CW (full) for walking. This initial assessment established a baseline for plantar pressure measurements. Subsequently, a systematic methodology was implemented, where 9 out of the 14 available inserts were removed one at a time to assess their impact on pressure distribution. The selected inserts for removal included Toe 1, Fore-Foot 1, Fore-Foot 2, Fore-Foot 3, Mid-Foot 1, Mid-Foot 2, Heel 1, Heel 4, and Heel. This strategic removal was crucial for obtaining specific plantar pressure values in each subcase across all participants, allowing for a focused analysis of how each insert contributed to overall pressure dynamics. It is important to note that the Toe 2 and Arch inserts were excluded from this removal process due to their consistently low-pressure measurements observed in both the standing and walking conditions. Despite their exclusion from the individual removal trials, pressure readings for these areas were still documented during the full insole assessments in both standing and walking trials. This approach ensured a comprehensive data set while also emphasizing the performance of the other inserts. Each participant completed a total of 10 thorough trials, which comprised one trial utilizing the complete insole and nine trials in which various inserts were removed under both standing (CS) and walking (CW) conditions. This extensive testing process enabled a robust analysis of the modular insole's performance. To ensure high accuracy and reliability in data collection, average pressure values, referred to as average zonal pressure (AZP), were recorded using the pressure-measuring insole in combination with a state-of-the-art running average algorithm. This approach not only enhanced the credibility of the results but also provided valuable insights into the effects of different insert configurations on plantar pressure, contributing to advancements in footwear design and foot care.

During the standing trials (CS), participants were instructed to maintain their natural upright posture for a duration of 5 s. This brief period was designed to capture baseline data on postural stability and weight distribution. In contrast, during the walking trials (CW), participants were asked to walk in a relaxed, unconstrained manner for a total of 20 s. This approach aimed to closely mimic real-world walking conditions, allowing for a more accurate assessment of the insole's effectiveness in practical scenarios. To evaluate the effectiveness of the modular insole design, researchers conducted a thorough analysis of the AZP values in the identified offloaded regions of the foot. This detailed analysis revealed significant reductions in pressure within targeted areas, which were expected to benefit from the insole's innovative design. The findings confirmed that the modular insole not only alleviated

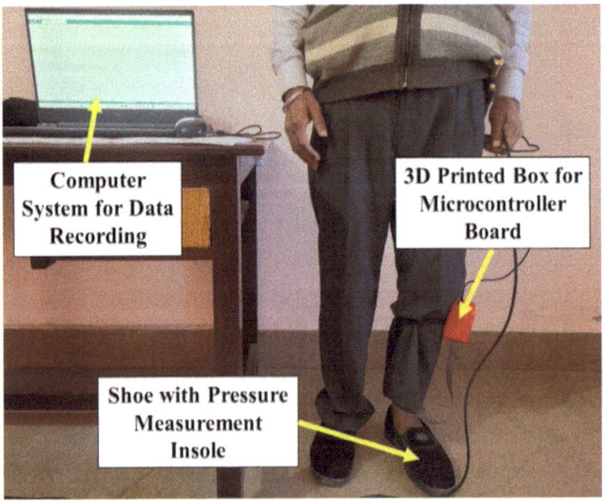

Fig. 8.1 Diabetic participant during trials with pressure-measuring insole and modular insole (inside the shoe). *Reproduced with permission from the Publisher* [3]

pressure but also showcased its potential to enhance overall comfort and performance in footwear, ultimately indicating its viability for improving user experience and promoting foot health in various activities.

8.3 Results

8.3.1 QUEST-Based Qualitative Analysis

In this comprehensive study assessing the effectiveness of insoles on user satisfaction, healthy participants showcased notable satisfaction levels. The QUEST score, a metric used to evaluate the comfort and functionality of the provided insoles, averaged 4.63 ± 0.08 for the HP-Q1 case and 4.61 ± 0.09 for the HP-Q2 case. These scores reflect a significant degree of approval from the healthy participants, indicating that they found the insoles well-designed and effective in meeting their comfort needs. Conversely, participants with diabetes reported even higher satisfaction levels, underscoring the insoles' impact on this particular group. The QUEST score for the DP-Q1 case reached an impressive 4.80 ± 0.06, suggesting that diabetic users not only found the insoles to be exceptionally comfortable but also felt that they addressed their specific health requirements effectively. The satisfaction continued to grow in the DP-Q2 case, where the score increased slightly to 4.81 ± 0.17. This consistent trend across different conditions suggests that the insoles are not only adaptable but also reliably beneficial for diabetic users. To enhance the understanding of these findings, Fig. 8.2 offers a comparative analysis of the QUEST scores pertaining to both healthy participants (Fig. 8.2a) and diabetic participants (Fig. 8.2b). This visual representation provides a deeper insight into the individual satisfaction levels and highlights both the similarities and differences in user experiences based on their health status. Overall, the data indicate that the insoles are highly valued across both demographic groups, with diabetic participants demonstrating particularly strong approval. This suggests that the design and functionality of the insoles could play a critical role in improving the quality of life for users, especially those managing diabetes. The findings emphasize the importance of tailored solutions in enhancing user satisfaction and well-being.

Based on the comprehensive findings from the QUEST assessment, participants indicated a high level of satisfaction with the performance of the modular insole, typically rating it between 4 and 5 on a scale of 1 to 5. These ratings not only reflect overall contentment but also signify a strong appreciation for both the design and functionality of the insole. In the qualitative trials, which encompassed a diverse group of participants, including healthy individuals (HP-Q1, HP-Q2) as well as individuals with diabetes (DP-Q1, DP-Q2), a range of feedback was collected regarding the insole's manufacturing quality and user experience. One significant observation was that participants did not notice the truncated areas located at Fore-Foot 1, Fore-Foot 2, Fore-Foot 3, Heel 1, and Heel 4 during the second qualitative trial (Q2), regardless

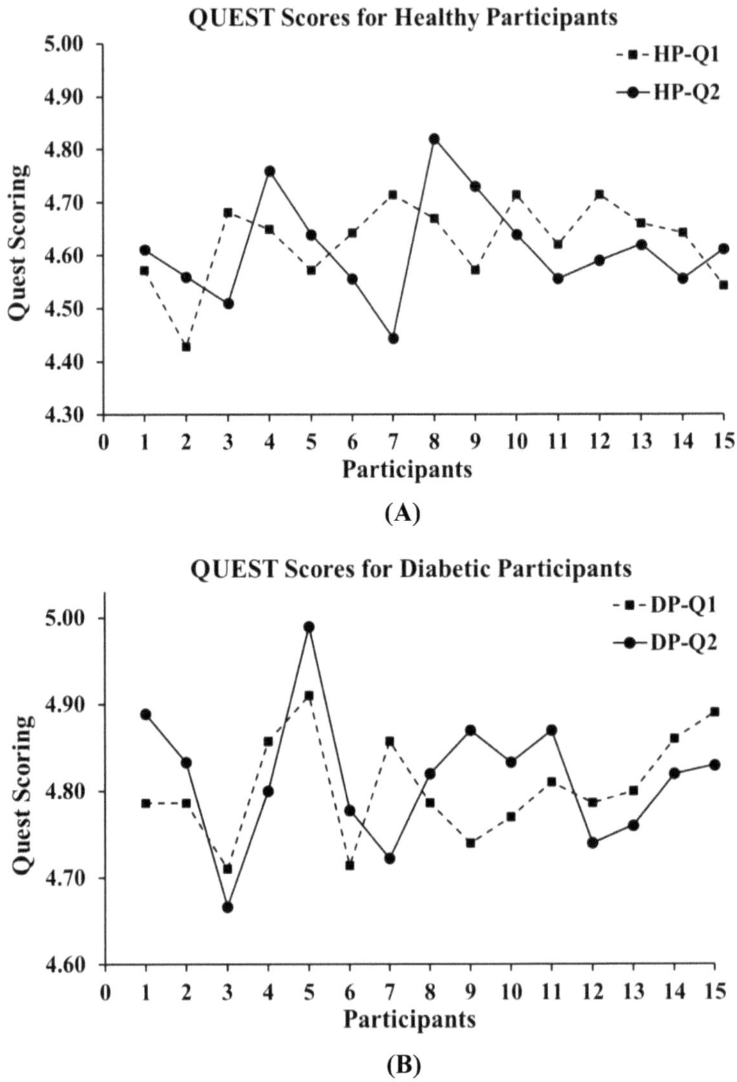

Fig. 8.2 QUEST scoring for: **a** Healthy participants and **b** Diabetic participants. *Reproduced with permission from the Publisher* [3]

of whether they were healthy (HP-Q2) or diabetic (DP-Q2). This lack of perception is likely due to the effective support provided by the surrounding surfaces of the insole, which appear to compensate for the truncated regions, thereby enhancing overall comfort and usability. Furthermore, participants reported that they only felt the voids created by the removal of inserts Toe 1 and Toe 2 when they actively engaged their toes. This indicates that, during regular use, the design effectively minimizes any negative impact on comfort, allowing for a seamless experience. The areas resulting from the removal of inserts Toe 3, Heel 2, and Heel 3 were found to be entirely unnoticeable, attributed to their small size, which further demonstrates the insole's thoughtful design. It is also important to note that the toe regions designated as Toe 3–5 did not significantly contribute to the overall plantar pressure values recorded during the trials. Consequently, these areas were excluded from the circular void design. This strategic decision was made to simplify the insole's structure while still ensuring it retained necessary functionality and comfort features. The overall feedback highlights the effectiveness of the insole's design in providing support and comfort for users with varying needs, affirming its potential for widespread application in the market.

The modular insole was designed with a streamlined process that ensured accessibility for all participants, regardless of their experience with footwear modifications. This user-friendly approach enables individuals to easily remove and reattach any insert from the mid-frame, ensuring that adjustments can be made without any hassle or confusion. Participants provided valuable feedback, consistently noting that the insole delivered an exceptional level of comfort, which highlighted its potential as an effective tool for enhancing foot health. The inserts can be tailored to meet specific needs, offering customizable support that adapts to various foot shapes and conditions. Furthermore, the positive responses from users were indicative of the insole's effectiveness, prompting recommendations for not only diabetic patients, who often face unique foot health challenges, but also for individuals who are at risk of developing nondiabetic foot ulceration. This broad application underscores the insole's versatility as a comfort solution, making it beneficial for a wider audience seeking to improve their overall foot health and comfort.

8.3.2 Evaluation of Pressure Offloading

As discussed earlier, a specialized pressure-mapping insole was designed and developed to measure plantar pressures with precision across eleven distinct segments of a modular insole. This innovative device was employed in a study involving two groups: healthy participants and individuals diagnosed with diabetes, allowing for a comparative analysis of foot pressure dynamics. The study was conducted under two specific conditions: standing and walking, which are essential activities that significantly affect foot pressure distribution. During the trials, comprehensive pressure data were gathered for each participant across both conditions. This data was then averaged to create a robust dataset, facilitating the calculation of AZP for each segment of the insole. The AZP values are critical in revealing the nuanced ways that pressure varies in different regions of the foot, helping researchers understand the implications of foot biomechanics in everyday activities. This in-depth analysis not only enriches our overall knowledge of how foot pressure is distributed, but it also plays a crucial role in identifying potential areas of concern, particularly in diabetic populations. Abnormal pressure distribution in these individuals can lead to serious complications, including ulcers and other foot-related health issues. By understanding these patterns, interventions can be tailored to mitigate risks and enhance foot health in at-risk populations.

Pressure Offloading for Healthy Participants

Table 8.2 offers a detailed summary of the AZP values, presented as mean ± standard deviation (S.D.), for nine distinct offloading scenarios evaluated in standing conditions among a group of healthy participants. This dataset includes measurements obtained both with the use of a full insole and in the absence of the insole, thereby facilitating a thorough comparison of offloading efficacy across the various conditions tested. In a similar way, Table 8.3 provides an extensive overview of the AZP values concerning plantar pressure offloading during walking conditions for the same cohort of healthy individuals. The analysis in Fig. 8.3 further examines the pressure values across multiple anatomical regions for healthy subjects engaged in both standing and walking scenarios. Throughout this study, pressure measurements were taken at eleven designated locations on the foot, of which nine were specifically targeted as offloaded sites to assess the effectiveness of the insole intervention. The corresponding AZP values, recorded in kilopascals (kPa), were gathered from a total of fifteen participants. These values were systematically averaged to produce a representative statistical landscape, expressed as mean ± S.D. This averaging process enhances the reliability of the findings by accounting for individual variability among participants. To provide a clearer visual representation, Fig. 8.3a and c displays the AZP values for healthy participants during both standing and walking conditions while utilizing the full modular insole. This insole system is designed for optimal performance, involving no removal of any inserts, which allows for a comprehensive evaluation of its impact on pressure distribution. Through this detailed analysis, the study aims to elucidate the effectiveness of the full insole in mitigating plantar pressure during different activities, contributing valuable insights to the field of orthopedic research and rehabilitation.

Figure 8.3b and d provides a detailed analysis of the AZP values recorded during trials where one insert was removed, illustrating the resultant offloading across various regions of the foot during both standing and walking conditions. In the standing condition utilizing the full insole, the data revealed that the maximum AZP occurred in the heel region, reaching a notable magnitude of 122.39 ± 3.62 kPa, as depicted in Fig. 8.3a. This significant pressure indicates the substantial load experienced by the heel during standing. Conversely, the arch region recorded the minimum AZP of only 3.86 ± 3.66 kPa. Of particular interest are the pressure magnitudes observed at the inserts for Toe 2 and the Arch, which were markedly low, accounting for just 1.83% and 0.76% of the total pressure recorded, respectively. Due to these minimal contributions to the overall pressure, the AZP values for Toe 2 and the Arch were deemed statistically insignificant for the study's objectives, suggesting that these regions might not require intense focus in terms of pressure alleviation strategies. Within the offloaded condition, illustrated in Fig. 8.3b, the plantar pressure values revealed a remarkable decrease. Specifically, reductions in pressure ranged from 97.52% at Mid-Foot 1 to an impressive 99.98% at Heel 1. This reduction signifies the effectiveness of the offloading measures employed during the trials, which

Table 8.2 AZP values (in kPa) for healthy participants (standing) in different offloading conditions. *Reproduced with permission from the Publisher* [3]

Removed inserts ↓	Toe 1	Toe 2	Fore-foot 1	Fore-foot 2	Fore-foot 3	Mid-foot 1	Mid-foot 2	Arch	Heel 1	Heel 4	Heel
No insole	63.52	7.40	98.34	24.35	78.66	32.27	25.73	3.09	116.64	17.77	133.44
Std. Dev	4.40	5.88	4.06	5.27	5.59	6.78	6.50	3.11	3.41	4.98	3.54
Full insole	47.52	9.20	73.74	18.55	54.82	22.67	23.55	3.86	105.96	19.31	122.39
Std. Dev	3.97	4.89	3.80	3.95	4.78	5.61	5.25	3.66	3.51	6.06	3.62
Toe 1 removed	3.52	10.53	74.78	31.87	42.41	21.26	24.45	3.17	95.50	12.08	82.82
Std. Dev	0.38	3.51	4.01	3.60	4.76	6.29	5.46	3.14	4.03	4.36	4.25
Fore-Foot 1 removed	51.86	25.22	4.89	18.73	87.51	50.05	60.60	3.53	98.93	44.23	147.58
Std. Dev	4.30	5.45	1.38	4.19	3.98	4.78	4.06	3.47	3.58	4.47	3.65
Fore-Foot 2 removed	34.71	9.19	53.13	3.31	66.95	22.47	40.72	3.59	115.28	30.70	148.95
Std. Dev	3.86	5.48	4.77	0.30	3.79	5.62	4.89	3.39	3.30	6.06	3.56
Fore-Foot 3 removed	84.69	20.10	87.35	15.28	3.82	15.59	19.22	13.18	86.16	23.30	144.67
Std. Dev	3.10	3.95	3.37	3.44	0.34	3.61	3.68	3.73	3.33	3.68	3.29
Mid-Foot 1 removed	67.52	21.29	88.78	16.40	47.05	3.97	34.81	4.06	109.65	42.74	141.72
Std. Dev	3.26	3.56	3.38	3.50	3.94	0.87	5.98	3.41	3.57	4.69	3.47
Mid-Foot 2 removed	55.69	41.65	34.16	29.71	91.86	60.48	4.41	3.47	117.52	33.77	155.36
Std. Dev	4.14	3.84	12.24	4.02	3.87	3.54	1.96	3.37	3.31	4.66	3.35

(continued)

Table 8.2 (continued)

Removed inserts ↓	Toe 1	Toe 2	Fore-foot 1	Fore-foot 2	Fore-foot 3	Mid-foot 1	Mid-foot 2	Arch	Heel 1	Heel 4	Heel
Heel 1 removed	46.71	5.97	111.58	40.03	89.06	29.83	27.35	10.85	3.86	58.52	115.08
Std. Dev	3.31	3.29	3.19	3.41	3.52	3.68	4.19	3.48	0.02	3.69	3.38
Heel 4 removed	46.71	5.97	111.58	40.03	89.06	29.83	27.35	10.85	58.52	3.09	115.08
Std. Dev	3.31	3.29	3.19	3.41	3.52	3.68	4.19	3.48	3.69	0.09	3.38
Heel removed	65.62	13.41	106.73	35.25	105.09	43.31	36.13	9.05	52.68	16.63	3.27
Std. Dev	4.36	5.12	3.72	4.34	4.01	4.35	3.58	6.01	5.52	4.28	0.50

* *Bold values represent the removed/offloaded inserts*

Table 8.3 AZP values (in kPa) for healthy participants (walking) in different offloading conditions. *Reproduced with permission from the Publisher* [3]

Removed inserts ↓	Toe 1	Toe 2	Fore-foot 1	Fore-foot 2	Fore-foot 3	Mid-foot 1	Mid-foot 2	Arch	Heel 1	Heel 4	Heel
No insole	67.16	6.55	114.50	30.53	69.23	22.26	21.64	4.60	116.88	19.58	138.43
Std. Dev	5.96	7.35	4.71	7.08	7.41	7.72	9.10	5.96	3.60	6.63	4.31
Full insole	128.10	17.06	171.69	93.98	201.21	78.32	80.87	22.32	143.63	48.66	195.16
Std. Dev	3.91	5.42	3.42	3.29	3.52	3.44	3.58	6.28	3.23	3.93	3.19
Toe 1 removed	3.33	17.79	80.88	36.58	163.14	103.99	106.44	3.19	104.56	71.88	195.55
Std. Dev	0.34	7.58	4.10	4.35	3.57	3.33	3.59	3.10	3.61	4.54	3.52
Fore-Foot 1 removed	77.12	21.64	4.36	52.35	192.36	85.48	102.29	10.03	130.71	71.09	186.05
Std. Dev	4.85	5.74	0.48	4.55	4.14	3.42	3.48	11.02	3.75	4.01	3.52
Fore-Foot 2 removed	130.07	58.66	150.93	4.07	122.55	62.83	87.95	3.26	97.04	50.44	150.24
Std. Dev	3.12	3.41	3.34	1.36	3.44	3.33	3.30	3.06	3.15	3.52	3.16
Fore-Foot 3 removed	132.77	40.54	32.36	57.86	5.70	45.55	63.84	15.02	123.82	55.21	171.36
Std. Dev	4.66	3.97	15.62	4.08	1.25	3.62	3.76	14.89	3.75	3.43	3.97
Mid-Foot 1 removed	129.03	16.72	171.36	88.96	196.58	3.51	67.99	15.07	140.75	47.41	193.46
Std. Dev	3.83	6.13	3.51	3.56	3.53	0.23	3.66	5.29	3.35	4.11	3.27
Mid-Foot 2 removed	92.42	25.12	118.24	27.95	71.85	55.48	3.43	11.89	128.78	59.29	170.78
Std. Dev	4.90	3.88	4.39	6.22	5.22	3.52	0.15	13.09	3.45	3.51	3.64

(continued)

Table 8.3 (continued)

Removed inserts ↓	Toe 1	Toe 2	Fore-foot 1	Fore-foot 2	Fore-foot 3	Mid-foot 1	Mid-foot 2	Arch	Heel 1	Heel 4	Heel
Heel 1 removed	93.55	77.55	92.07	58.93	233.12	121.44	115.74	3.27	3.83	79.89	182.08
Std. Dev	4.63	3.26	9.22	5.63	3.12	3.41	3.45	3.23	0.45	3.87	3.35
Heel 4 removed	75.79	15.84	159.45	85.37	167.68	69.96	73.07	12.21	133.69	3.55	193.68
Std. Dev	3.38	4.02	3.13	3.13	3.08	3.32	3.25	3.36	3.13	0.26	3.11
Heel removed	68.02	22.30	125.31	50.83	132.90	71.30	44.75	6.58	28.67	11.93	3.57
Std. Dev	4.52	7.71	4.15	4.58	4.12	4.22	4.56	7.10	3.50	4.03	0.31

* *Bold values represent the removed/offloaded inserts*

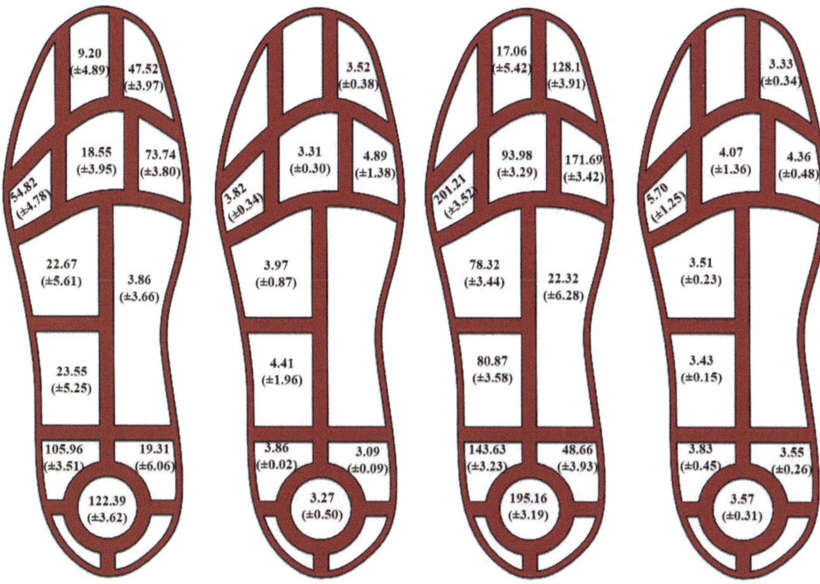

Fig. 8.3 AZP values (in kPa, mean ± S.D.) for healthy participants: **a** Full insole with all inserts during standing, **b** Offloading of regions by removing their respective insert in standing position, **c** Full insole with all inserts during walking, **d** Offloading of regions by removing their respective insert in walking condition. *Reproduced with permission from the Publisher* [3]

aimed to distribute pressure more evenly across the foot. The maximum AZP value in this offloaded scenario was observed at Fore-Foot 1, measuring 4.89 ± 1.38 kPa. This value reinforces the efficacy of the offloading process, highlighting how it successfully lowered pressure in key regions during standing conditions across all participants involved in the study. Overall, this data emphasizes the critical importance of optimizing insole design and strategic offloading approaches. Such enhancements are essential not only for alleviating undue pressure on high-risk plantar regions but also for improving overall foot health and comfort.

Figure 8.3c provides a detailed representation of the AZP values measured in healthy participants utilizing full insoles during walking activities. The data collected across various regions of the foot highlights critical differences in pressure distribution. Notably, the heel region demonstrated the highest AZP, with a value of 195.16 ± 3.19 kPa. This elevated pressure in the heel is particularly important, as it indicates a focal point of stress during walking, which can place this area at a higher risk for skin breakdown and injuries, such as pressure ulcers. In contrast, the arch region exhibited significantly lower AZP, recorded at just 22.32 ± 6.28 kPa. This finding suggests that the arch plays a lesser role in supporting weight and distributing pressure compared to the heel. Understanding these variations in AZP is crucial for developing effective strategies to mitigate the risk of foot injuries. Areas experiencing higher pressure are more susceptible to skin damage, while regions with lower pressure typically present a diminished risk. Additionally, it is noteworthy that the AZP values observed at the inserts labeled Toe 2 and Arch were minimal, accounting for only 1.44% and 1.88% of the total recorded pressure, respectively. Given their negligible contributions to the overall pressure profile, the decision to exclude these inserts from further evaluation was made. Their removal is unlikely to significantly influence the outcomes of the trials, emphasizing the focus on more impactful areas of concern in pressure management during walking. This nuanced understanding of foot pressure dynamics is essential for designing interventions aimed at preventing pressure-related injuries in various populations.

Additionally, Fig. 8.3d presents a comprehensive overview of the AZP values observed during cases involving pressure offloading. The data reveals a striking reduction in pressure across various foot segments, with decreases ranging from 92.71% at the Heel 4 segment to an impressive 98.17% at the Heel segment. This substantial alleviation of pressure is particularly noteworthy, yet it is important to highlight that the highest pressure experienced during the offloading phase was recorded at the Fore-Foot 3 segment, which demonstrated an AZP value of 5.70 ± 1.25 kPa. Following this, the pressures observed at the Fore-Foot 1 and Fore-Foot 2 segments were also elevated, measuring 4.36 ± 0.48 kPa and 4.07 ± 1.36 kPa, respectively. Although these pressures may seem relatively minor when compared to the significantly higher initial heel pressure, they signify vital contact points that come into play during the heel strike phase of walking. This emphasizes the importance of the Heel, Heel 4, and Heel 1 segments in understanding foot dynamics and optimizing footwear design. Following an extensive analysis of the collected data and the incorporation of participant feedback, we concluded that the modular insole design effectively facilitated adequate pressure offloading across all nine targeted regions of the foot. The range of pressure reduction observed, between 92.71% and 98.17%, underscores the effectiveness of the insole in promoting overall foot health and preventing potential injuries during walking activities. This thorough assessment contributes significantly to our understanding of how strategic pressure offloading can dramatically mitigate the risks associated with prolonged standing and walking. This is particularly relevant for individuals who are at an elevated risk of developing foot-related complications, thus highlighting the importance of innovative solutions in enhancing comfort and health in everyday mobility.

Pressure Offloading for Diabetic Participants

The recorded AZP values, presented as mean ± standard deviation, for the 15 diabetic participants were collected under both standing and walking conditions, as detailed in Tables 8.4 and 8.5. The study examined two scenarios: the first involved the use of a full insole, while the second examined the participants without an insole, facilitating a comprehensive comparative analysis of how each scenario affected pressure offloading. In the standing position, participants wearing the full insole demonstrated the highest AZP in the heel region, which peaked at 40.92 ± 12.45 kPa, as illustrated in Fig. 4a. This finding emphasizes the concentration of pressure in the heel area, commonly associated with weight-bearing activities. Conversely, the arch region exhibited the lowest AZP, with a mean value of just 4.88 ± 4.53 kPa. These values are particularly revealing when contextualized against the findings in healthy participants, where the pressure readings at the insert locations, specifically Toe 2 and the Arch, remained remarkably low, accounting for only 2.78% and 2.19% of the total pressure distribution, respectively. Due to their minimal impact, these regions were classified as inconsequential and were subsequently excluded from the offloading trials, streamlining the focus to more impactful zones. In terms of the effectiveness of offloading, a substantial reduction in AZP values was observed. The most notable decreases were recorded, showing a reduction of 87.11% at the Fore-Foot 3 region and an impressive 97.82% at Heel 1, as depicted in Fig. 8.4b. These reductions highlight the efficacy of the full insole in evenly redistributing pressure across the plantar surface, thereby mitigating risk and potentially preventing complications associated with excessive pressure, such as ulcerations or other injuries. Overall, these findings underscore the importance of strategic insole use in managing and alleviating pressure for diabetic patients, promoting better foot health and mobility.

The AZP values measured for diabetic participants while walking, as illustrated in Fig. 8.4c, highlighted noteworthy findings regarding pressure distribution across various foot regions. The heel region recorded the highest pressure, at an average of 130.96 ± 4.27 kPa, underscoring the significant load that this area endures during walking. This elevation in pressure is particularly concerning for diabetic individuals, as it can lead to an increased risk of skin breakdown and subsequent ulceration. In contrast, the arch region demonstrated markedly lower AZP, quantified at just 12.45 ± 9.51 kPa. This significant difference highlights the varying mechanical stresses experienced in different areas of the foot. The plantar region exhibited higher AZP values, indicating a potential risk zone that warrants careful monitoring and management, especially in diabetic patients who may have compromised circulation and skin integrity. Furthermore, similar to findings from the standing condition, AZP values recorded at the insert locations, specifically, Toe 2 and the Arch, were minimal, contributing a mere 2.21% and 2.06% of total pressure, respectively. This minimal contribution supports the rationale for their exclusion from the offloading analyses, as their impact on overall foot pressure is negligible. Figure 8.4d presents the results of the pressure offloading trials, demonstrating a significant reduction in pressure across various foot segments while walking. The pressure reduction achieved remarkable levels, ranging from 81.52% at the segment labeled Heel 4 to an impressive 97.19% at the heel region itself. These results strongly affirm the effectiveness of the full insole in alleviating pressure points on the foot of diabetic participants during dynamic activities, which is crucial for preventing pressure-related complications and enhancing overall foot health. Moving forward, these insights will be valuable for developing strategies aimed at improving foot care for individuals with diabetes.

Table 8.4 AZP values (in kPa) for participants with diabetes (standing) in different offloading conditions. *Reproduced with permission from the Publisher* [3]

Removed inserts ↓	Toe 1	Toe 2	Fore-foot 1	Fore-foot 2	Fore-foot 3	Mid-foot 1	Mid-foot 2	Arch	Heel 1	Heel 4	Heel
No insole	26.07	3.26	40.00	16.83	41.78	10.40	8.64	3.09	29.26	5.10	57.77
Std. Dev	9.64	3.33	16.48	7.74	9.37	6.34	6.50	3.06	6.62	4.21	7.17
Full insole	24.40	6.19	33.43	24.34	30.74	13.63	17.89	4.88	47.40	15.23	67.92
Std. Dev	9.37	5.24	11.69	6.63	9.37	8.37	8.45	4.53	9.99	5.69	12.45
Toe 1 removed	2.42	14.88	90.12	37.40	80.62	24.33	26.39	4.23	118.69	12.53	104.10
Std. Dev	2.46	4.18	7.63	5.25	6.03	7.43	8.26	4.63	5.73	5.74	10.12
Fore-Foot 1 removed	56.85	19.09	3.74	23.63	115.56	45.61	66.93	3.75	84.53	36.64	125.87
Std. Dev	3.76	4.88	1.66	3.72	4.11	5.41	4.50	3.55	3.73	4.55	3.45
Fore-Foot 2 removed	38.24	8.43	14.39	2.47	76.49	16.93	32.95	3.68	102.99	16.25	123.96
Std. Dev	3.33	3.21	3.38	0.53	3.28	3.38	3.41	3.19	3.12	3.62	3.28
Fore-Foot 3 removed	70.68	13.30	57.66	12.93	3.96	14.91	18.94	9.14	90.81	23.65	152.14
Std. Dev	3.98	6.03	5.81	4.38	0.38	3.85	3.95	5.88	3.39	3.60	3.28
Mid-Foot 1 removed	62.18	18.64	84.40	16.59	57.46	1.10	51.84	3.95	118.96	56.87	153.89
Std. Dev	3.14	3.22	3.24	3.17	3.30	0.08	3.11	3.17	3.26	3.23	3.14
Mid-Foot 2 removed	90.81	24.42	116.27	27.32	69.96	53.77	2.26	12.32	126.54	57.33	172.35
Std. Dev	4.76	3.85	4.56	6.27	5.39	3.47	0.06	13.99	3.47	3.55	3.70

(continued)

Table 8.4 (continued)

Removed inserts ↓	Toe 1	Toe 2	Fore-foot 1	Fore-foot 2	Fore-foot 3	Mid-foot 1	Mid-foot 2	Arch	Heel 1	Heel 4	Heel
Heel 1 removed	67.83	3.60	122.84	18.34	73.24	16.82	16.53	3.14	1.03	7.72	83.44
Std. Dev	4.16	3.57	3.92	4.47	4.30	4.37	4.25	3.11	0.02	4.11	4.27
Heel 4 removed	42.63	11.02	81.93	29.09	61.90	42.73	32.58	7.61	68.93	1.58	106.83
Std. Dev	3.34	3.26	3.25	3.14	3.21	3.32	4.15	3.31	3.27	0.37	3.37
Heel removed	27.76	11.44	54.96	15.17	19.14	11.41	14.02	3.08	60.15	6.55	3.09
Std. Dev	3.56	3.39	3.50	3.49	3.60	3.97	3.83	3.08	3.32	3.46	0.32

* *Bold values represent the removed/offloaded inserts*

Table 8.5 AZP values (in kPa) for participants with diabetes (walking) in different offloading conditions. *Reproduced with permission from the Publisher* [3]

Removed inserts ↓	Toe 1	Toe 2	Fore-foot 1	Fore-foot 2	Fore-foot 3	Mid-foot 1	Mid-foot 2	Arch	Heel 1	Heel 4	Heel
No insole	7.75	5.51	28.68	17.20	14.71	13.45	18.07	3.07	89.63	35.84	105.68
Std. Dev	3.50	3.47	4.00	3.63	3.98	3.61	3.64	3.07	3.23	3.31	3.13
Full insole	55.76	13.35	66.20	37.13	72.20	49.66	40.25	12.45	98.84	27.07	130.96
Std. Dev	6.74	5.26	9.01	6.73	8.18	4.84	6.38	9.51	4.25	6.40	4.27
Toe 1 removed	3.44	10.84	62.83	44.17	111.20	31.62	44.12	3.62	93.55	25.18	114.42
Std. Dev	0.27	6.27	5.23	4.39	4.29	7.50	5.05	3.44	3.60	4.85	3.42
Fore-Foot 1 removed	88.05	23.22	4.32	61.19	216.91	87.55	105.50	12.18	138.52	78.71	188.00
Std. Dev	4.35	5.88	0.52	3.42	3.29	3.39	3.42	11.06	3.58	3.41	3.55
Fore-Foot 2 removed	101.82	27.17	75.74	6.86	70.55	39.88	29.44	8.95	137.52	44.20	112.35
Std. Dev	4.96	3.61	5.54	1.44	6.87	3.68	5.20	13.51	3.41	3.80	5.60
Fore-Foot 3 removed	90.17	17.42	70.66	24.43	5.66	23.10	21.88	8.51	111.64	31.09	114.06
Std. Dev	4.53	5.67	5.30	4.86	1.11	4.15	3.51	6.38	3.69	4.27	4.37
Mid-Foot 1 removed	65.98	25.61	32.42	25.58	26.23	4.32	18.54	3.14	128.29	11.99	107.97
Std. Dev	3.92	5.60	4.19	8.88	5.14	0.57	3.87	3.15	3.76	5.87	3.64
Mid-Foot 2 removed	163.14	35.49	176.90	77.94	127.77	76.46	3.52	23.70	139.88	71.48	180.34
Std. Dev	3.45	3.46	3.51	3.25	3.57	3.75	0.28	16.23	3.36	3.21	3.84

(continued)

Table 8.5 (continued)

Removed inserts ↓	Toe 1	Toe 2	Fore-foot 1	Fore-foot 2	Fore-foot 3	Mid-foot 1	Mid-foot 2	Arch	Heel 1	Heel 4	Heel
Heel 1 removed	139.47	21.16	156.73	80.90	159.99	72.74	71.58	5.86	3.58	36.24	153.71
Std. Dev	3.67	7.41	3.79	3.95	4.37	3.39	3.50	6.09	0.31	4.86	4.00
Heel 4 removed	113.38	28.53	122.55	41.19	92.60	43.17	38.77	7.45	97.71	3.19	110.94
Std. Dev	3.59	5.24	3.84	4.82	3.49	4.25	3.61	3.78	3.41	0.08	3.32
Heel removed	48.68	8.43	131.26	50.21	139.47	54.02	39.03	17.64	32.80	16.05	3.67
Std. Dev	3.60	3.39	3.45	3.59	3.35	3.61	3.63	4.05	3.55	3.70	0.54

* *Bold values represent the removed/offloaded inserts*

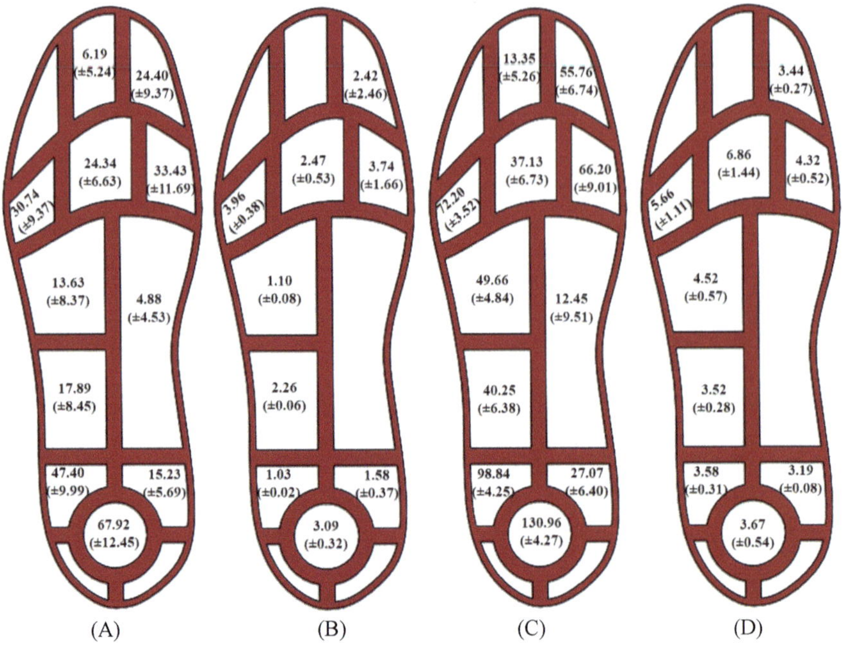

Fig. 8.4 AZP values (in kPa, mean ± S.D.) for diabetic participants: **a** Full insole with all inserts during standing, **b** Offloading of regions by removing their respective insert in standing position, **c** Full insole with all inserts during walking, **d** Offloading of regions by removing their respective insert in walking condition. *Reproduced with permission from the Publisher* [3]

8.4 Discussion

After conducting a comprehensive analysis of the results obtained from both healthy and diabetic participants, several noteworthy observations emerged about the influence of a modular insole on pressure distribution during various activities. Firstly, it was revealed that diabetic participants exhibited significantly lower AZP values while using the full insole when compared to their healthy counterparts. This pattern was consistent in both standing and walking conditions, highlighting the unique challenges faced by individuals with diabetes. In the standing position, the maximum AZP values were predominantly concentrated in the heel region, which is critical for weight-bearing. Healthy participants demonstrated a mean AZP of 122.39 ± 3.62 kPa, indicating a higher level of pressure in this area. In contrast, diabetic participants recorded a markedly lower mean AZP of 67.92 ± 12.45 kPa, suggesting their inability to distribute weight effectively through the heel. This disparity in pressure can likely be attributed to potential complications associated with diabetes, such as neuropathy and decreased circulation. Similarly, during walking, the trend persisted, with healthy participants exhibiting a maximum AZP of 195.16 ± 3.19 kPa in the heel region, which emphasizes their superior ability to absorb and distribute impact forces. Diabetic participants, however, showed a maximum AZP of only 130.96 ± 4.27 kPa in the same region, indicating compromised biomechanics while walking. Moreover, the analysis extended to the forefoot regions, namely Fore-Foot 1, Fore-Foot 2, and Fore-Foot 3, which demonstrated comparable patterns of pressure distribution across both groups. This consistency in pressure values points to the overarching impact of diabetes, which often alters the structural integrity of the foot, particularly the stiffness of the plantar fascia. The changes in the plantar fascia can lead to swelling and discomfort, causing diabetic individuals to avoid placing their entire foot adequately while standing and walking. In summary, these findings underline the importance of understanding how diabetes affects foot mechanics and pressure distribution, ultimately emphasizing the need for targeted interventions, such as the implementation of specialized insoles, to enhance comfort and mobility for diabetic individuals [6, 7].

The study's findings revealed that the AZP values remained consistently similar across all nine offloading conditions tested, involving both healthy and diabetic participants, during both standing and walking activities. This remarkable consistency underscores the effectiveness of the modular insole in providing adequate pressure relief and support, indicating its reliability across a variety of conditions. Moreover, the QUEST results highlighted that diabetic participants reported the modular insole as a comfortable and reliable solution for their walking and pressure-offloading needs. This positive feedback was further reaffirmed by the measured offloading values, which were recorded during both standing and walking scenarios across the nine different cases involving diabetic individuals. These results underscore the practical benefits of the insole, demonstrating its ability to function effectively in everyday situations. Importantly, it should be noted that the heel region of the foot is particularly prone to ulceration in diabetic patients due to factors like impaired circulation and neuropathy. The modular insole addresses this concern by redistributing and significantly reducing pressure in this vulnerable area, making it an essential tool for foot health management in individuals with diabetes. By taking proactive measures to address these risks, the use of the modular insole can enhance foot safety and overall quality of life for diabetic patients, ultimately promoting better health outcomes and preventing severe complications associated with foot ulcers.

8.5 Conclusions

In conclusion, the innovative modular insole has proven to be highly effective in relieving pressure on the foot's plantar fascia, a crucial aspect for individuals who suffer from diabetic ulcers. These ulcers often arise due to the increased stress and strain on specific areas of the foot, making effective pressure redistribution essential for promoting healing. The modular design of the insole allows for a customizable fit, accommodating various foot shapes and sizes, which can further enhance comfort and support. By redistributing pressure away from the sensitive plantar region, the modular insole not only alleviates pain but also significantly improves overall mobility and quality of life for individuals facing diabetic foot complications. The findings from this study shed light on the intricate mechanisms that contribute to ulceration in diabetic foot, providing valuable insights that can guide both research and clinical practice [8–11]. For healthcare providers, the implementation of the modular insole presents a proactive approach to preventing the progression of foot ulcers. By addressing pressure points effectively, these insoles can play a vital role in reducing the risk of serious complications, including infections and amputations, which can arise when ulcers are left untreated. This understanding underscores the importance of incorporating effective footwear solutions like the modular insole into diabetes management strategies, ultimately leading to better patient outcomes and enhanced foot health.

References

1. Chanda A, Unnikrishnan V (2018) Novel insole design for diabetic foot ulcer management. Proc Inst Mech Eng Part H J Eng Med. 232, 1182–1195
2. Singh G, Chanda A (2024) Finite element modeling of diabetic foot: a state-of-the-art review. Eng Res Express 6:012507
3. Singh G, Bose D, Chanda A (2025) Development and testing of a novel diabetic orthosis for plantar pressure reduction. Facta Univ Ser Mech Eng. https://doi.org/10.22190/FUME240725044S
4. Fu JCM, Chen YJ, Li CF, Hsiao YH, Chen CH (2022) The effect of three dimensional printing hinged ankle foot orthosis for equinovarus control in stroke patients. Clin Biomech 94:105622
5. Burger H et al (2019) Cross-cultural adaptation and Rasch validation of the Slovene version of the Orthotics and Prosthetics Users' Survey (OPUS) Client Satisfaction with Device (CSD) in upper-limb prosthesis users. Ann Phys Rehabil Med 62:168–173
6. Singh G, Lamba A, Chanda A (2024) Role of additive manufacturing for the management of diabetic foot ulcers. In Addit Manuf Biomed Appl 19–38 (Springer, Singapore). https://doi.org/10.1007/978-981-97-5456-4_2
7. Bose D, Singh G, Gupta S, Chanda A (2024) Development of a novel customized insole for effective pressure offloading in diabetic patients. Prosthesis 6:341–356
8. Gupta S et al (2023) Diabot: development of a diabetic foot pressure tracking device. J 6, 32–47
9. Chhikara K, Singh G, Gupta S, Chanda A (2022) Progress of additive manufacturing in fabrication of foot orthoses for diabetic patients: A review. Ann 3D Print Med 8, 100085
10. Singh G, Gupta S, Chanda A (2021) Biomechanical modelling of diabetic foot ulcers: A computational study. J Biomech 127:110699
11. Gupta S, Singh G, Chanda A (2021) Prediction of diabetic foot ulcer progression: a computational study. Biomed Phys Eng Express 7:065020

Chapter 9
Summary, Limitations, and Future Work

9.1 Summary

Diabetic foot complications present a significant global health challenge, posing extensive medical, economic, and social burdens on affected individuals and their families. One of the most prevalent of these complications is diabetic foot ulcers (DFUs), which can lead to a cascade of severe health issues such as infections, lower limb amputations, and even increased mortality rates. The persistence of DFUs, despite recent advancements in medical technology and treatment methodologies, highlights an ongoing crisis and underscores the urgent need for innovative strategies focused on prevention and management [1, 2]. Current evidence indicates that the prevalence of DFUs remains alarmingly high, which calls for a focused research effort. There are limited studies that delve into the biomechanics of the diabetic foot and strategies for ulcer prevention [3–5]. This represents a critical area requiring attention, as understanding the mechanical dynamics of the foot could lead to more effective intervention strategies. Chapter 1 of this book presents the motivation behind the study of DFUs by emphasizing their significance not only in clinical contexts but also within the broader spectrum of public health. It articulates a clear problem statement that highlights the complexities and multifactorial challenges associated with biomechanical modeling of these ulcers. This chapter also identifies several key research gaps in the existing methodologies and approaches, advocating for a more comprehensive understanding of the biomechanical forces at play. By addressing these critical aspects, the chapter seeks to lay a solid foundation for future research endeavors and clinical practices aimed at improving management strategies for DFUs. In Chap. 2, a comprehensive literature review on the biomechanics of foot structure is presented, elucidating how variations in anatomical features can significantly influence overall foot mechanics and functionality. The chapter discusses the progression of current computational models developed to predict and analyze the development of DFUs, critically examining their effectiveness and limitations within clinical settings. Moreover, various medical interventions

A. Chanda and G. Singh, *Diabetic Foot Ulcer*, Biomedical Materials for Multi-functional Applications, https://doi.org/10.1007/978-981-95-2484-6_9

and clinical practices currently in use for the prevention and treatment of DFUs are thoroughly explored.

Chapter 3 delves into the intricate biomechanical modeling of diabetic ulcers, specifically examining the differences across varying foot types, namely the normal arch and flatfoot. In this study, we developed detailed computational models that accurately replicate the anatomical structures and functional behaviors of these foot types. This approach allows us to evaluate how mechanical stresses differ between them under various conditions. To investigate the risk of ulcer formation, we examined a diverse range of ulcer diameters and depths. Our analysis was designed to assess how these parameters influence plantar stresses, ultimately paving the way for a clearer understanding of the mechanical environment that prompts individuals to ulceration. By quantifying the resultant data, we not only enhanced our comprehension of the underlying biomechanics but also aimed to inform more effective preventive strategies for diabetic patients who are at heightened risk for foot ulcers. Building on the findings from Chaps. 3, 4 expands the scope of our research to include biomechanical modeling of diabetic ulcers at all potential locations on the foot. This chapter highlights the importance of understanding where ulcers are likely to develop and how their progression may vary by location. We conducted a thorough investigation into the pressure distribution patterns characteristic of each ulcer site, revealing how these patterns can substantially influence the risk of ulceration. In addition to the biomechanical assessments, the chapter discusses the clinical implications of ulcer location in comprehensive detail. Recognizing how the unique mechanical stresses at different sites contribute to ulcer formation can significantly enhance clinical interventions. Our work culminates in the development of prediction models that aid healthcare professionals in formulating tailored prevention and treatment plans. These plans emphasize a personalized approach, taking into account the specific mechanical profiles and risks associated with each patient's foot type and ulcer location, ultimately improving the management of DFUs. The findings in Chap. 5 present a novel finite element modeling approach to analyze realistic wound geometries and the associated stresses and strains during skin healing. Unlike prior work limited to standard wound shapes, this research examines a variety of wound types, including diabetic, venous, pressure, and ulcer wounds, under natural skin tension across healing phases. The findings offer valuable insights for pre-surgical planning and robotic-assisted wound closure, aiming to prevent tissue overstrain and improve healing outcomes. Chapter 6 emphasizes the imperative need for ongoing technological advancements within the field with the overarching goal of improving patient outcomes and mitigating the complications associated with diabetic foot conditions. Through this detailed exploration, the work aims to enhance the understanding of DFU complexities and foster innovative solutions that could lead to better clinical results.

Chapter 7 discussed the development of an innovative smart pressure-measuring insole that employs force-sensing resistors (FSRs) to continuously monitor and record real-time plantar pressure during experimental trials. This state-of-the-art technology allows for detailed data collection and analysis, offering valuable insights into the effectiveness of the modular system in alleviating pressure on targeted areas of the foot. By understanding these pressure dynamics, researchers can assess how well the insole performs in real-world scenarios. Moreover, this chapter outlines the design and engineering of a novel modular insole specifically aimed at offloading plantar pressure for individuals living with diabetes. The integration of the modular offloading insole with the smart pressure-measuring insole was a crucial step for a forthcoming clinical study, which aimed to investigate the capacity of the modular insole to effectively off-load pressure and prevent potential injuries. Chapter 8 presents the findings from the clinical validation of the developed modular insole, with a specific focus on its ability to off-load plantar pressure in patients who are at risk of developing DFUs, an unfortunately common complication for those with diabetes. To evaluate the insole's effectiveness, a comprehensive and rigorous comparative study was conducted involving diverse groups of participants, including both healthy individuals and diabetic patients. The data collected was both quantitative, measuring pressure alterations, and qualitative, providing feedback from participants regarding their experiences while using the insole. The outcomes of the clinical trials were promising, revealing that the modular insole significantly reduced peak pressures in high-risk areas of the foot when compared to traditional offloading insoles. This substantial reduction in pressure is critical, as it plays a pivotal role in preventing the onset of DFUs, which can result in severe complications and impact the quality of life for individuals with diabetes. In this chapter presented the summary, limitations, and future scope of the work, stating that the findings presented are expected to be instrumental in developing tailored interventions, such as custom orthotics, aimed at managing and preventing DFUs effectively. These insights may contribute to improved patient care and outcomes for those at risk, underscoring the importance of ongoing innovation in the field of diabetes management.

9.2 Limitations

9.2.1 Computational Models

There are several limitations of this work that should be acknowledged. Firstly, the foot was modeled as a single entity with uniform isotropic mechanical properties. While this simplified approach provided reasonable accuracy for simulations concerning diabetic foot properties, the incorporation of a more intricate model that includes distinct tissues, such as skin, fat, and various types of bone, could significantly enhance the fidelity of the results. A detailed geometrical model generated through advanced techniques like 3D scanning or image segmentation could yield insights into the relative plantar stresses that reflect a higher degree of accuracy, capturing the complexities of the anatomical structures involved. Secondly, it is important to recognize that foot sizes and plantar contours vary considerably across different patients. This variability can influence the outcomes of the simulations, as the unique biomechanical characteristics of each individual's foot can alter force distributions. While the general qualitative trends observed in this research are expected to hold true across diverse foot and ulcer geometries, future studies that systematically account for these individual differences may lead to improvements in the precision of quantitative results. Thirdly, the phenomenon of swelling associated with DFUs was not incorporated into our current model. Swelling can significantly alter the foot-floor contact area, thereby affecting stress distribution in the vicinity of the ulcers. This change has the potential to shield the ulcer wall from stress, with the extent of this shielding being contingent on the size and distribution of the swollen tissue. Although this could impact the calculated maximum stresses, it is unlikely to drastically change the identified locations of peak ulcer wall stress. Future research that explores the effects of varying degrees of swelling on diabetic foot stress could contribute to a more precise understanding of these dynamics. Lastly, it is essential to consider that diabetic ulcers present with a diverse range of shapes and depths [6, 7]. In this work, we focused exclusively on modeling ulcers with a standard circular geometry and uniform depth to isolate the impact of ulcer location. However, actual diabetic ulcers often exhibit noncircular forms and varying depths, which can be accurately assessed through clinical measurement techniques. In summary, acknowledging these limitations and addressing them in future investigations will enhance the overall robustness of the findings and contribute to a better understanding of the mechanical factors influencing DFUs.

We utilized a straightforward maximum stress-based criterion to evaluate ulcer progression, recognizing the complexity involved in such assessments. The literature presents various damage models designed to analyze and quantify tissue damage in a more precise manner. For instance, Maghami et al. [8] explored the impact of diabetes on crack growth trajectories in human cortical bone through a phase field fracture model. Their research highlighted the significant role of material heterogeneity, particularly the microstructural features of the bone, and the intrinsic interactions between cracks and surrounding microstructures, which collectively contribute to the overall fragility of bone under diabetic conditions. Similarly, Saez et al. [9] formulated an anisotropic multi-scale damage model aimed at characterizing the progressive rupture of fibrous soft tissues. This model was rigorously tested through finite element modeling on blood vessels following angioplasty, showcasing its utility in real-world medical scenarios. Bates and Ma [10] further delved into the phenomenon of progressive rupture within a soft tissue stress relaxation model. Their research simulated isolated micro-yield events that occurred in sequence throughout the tissue, emphasizing how interactions with adjacent regions, as well as the material's anisotropic characteristics, could significantly influence the overall yielding behavior of the tissue.

Li [11] provided a comprehensive review of a range of isotropic and anisotropic soft tissue damage models, specifically focusing on their application to human arteries. This review encompassed various approaches, including deterministic and probabilistic damage models, as well as microstructure-based damage models, thus linking the concepts of damage and fracture. The insights gained from employing such advanced models can lead to more accurate assessments of damage severity and ulcer progression. Looking ahead, there is a need to incorporate more intricate foot models that account for inner anatomical structures, diverse ulcer geometries, and other relevant variables. Addressing the limitations of previous studies by expanding the scope of analysis may yield significantly more accurate and clinically relevant results. In summary, this study marks a pioneering effort to analyze how ulcer location affects diabetic plantar stresses and to develop predictive formulations for ulcer growth and the emergence of new ulcerations across different standard foot sizes. This essential knowledge is crucial for healthcare professionals, as it enhances their ability to assess foot ulcers effectively and implement timely, targeted interventions for their patients.

9.2.2 Developed Intervention

It is important to acknowledge certain limitations associated with the design and functionality of the modular diabetic insole to enhance its effectiveness and user experience. A comprehensive analysis of the average zonal pressure (AZP) values gathered from the heel region, particularly at the ball of the foot, highlights that the heel consistently maintains significant contact with the shoe during the heel-striking phase of walking. This persistent contact suggests that the current design of the insole may not optimally distribute pressure across the foot. As a result, users may experience discomfort or face potential issues related to improper foot mechanics, which could lead to complications such as blisters, calluses, or even more severe foot injuries over time. To address this concern, one viable solution would be to decrease the radius of the silicone insert specifically in the heel region. By implementing this change, we would effectively increase the overall surface area of heel inserts 1 through 4. This adjustment is crucial as it could significantly enhance the comfort experienced by the user by facilitating better pressure distribution across the foot. Improved pressure distribution would not only support the foot's natural mechanics during walking but could also promote a healthier gait pattern, ultimately reducing the risk of foot-related complications that individuals with diabetes often face. Furthermore, it is crucial that trials involving the modular insole, particularly those related to walking, are conducted over an extended timeframe. Prolonged evaluation periods will yield valuable insights into the insole's performance attributes, overall comfort levels, and its adaptability to the individual's foot structure and walking style over time. Such comprehensive testing is essential to identify any long-term effects and variations in performance, which can inform further refinements and enhancements. By gathering detailed data from these prolonged trials, researchers and designers will be better equipped to make informed modifications to the product, ultimately enhancing the efficacy, comfort, and user satisfaction of the modular diabetic insole for long-term use. This iterative process of design and testing will ensure the insole meets the specific needs of its users, fostering better foot health and mobility [12–14].

This study aims to provide significant benefits to diabetic patients by delivering a comprehensive analysis of plantar pressure dynamics. Understanding these dynamics is crucial because they play a central role in both preventing the formation of foot ulcers and managing their recurrence, conditions that can lead to serious complications and greatly impact a patient's quality of life. The research specifically investigates how variations in plantar pressure affect diabetic individuals, leading to increased risk factors for ulceration. By examining these variations in detail, we can identify specific pressure points and conditions that elevate the likelihood of foot injuries and ulcers. This understanding is essential for developing targeted interventions that can mitigate these risks. Furthermore, the study focuses on the need for both accessible and innovative solutions tailored to effectively manage DFUs. Current treatment options can be limited, and many patients may struggle to access the necessary care. By highlighting these challenges, the research emphasizes the importance of enhancing patient care and support systems. The development and implementation of new strategies, such as advanced monitoring technologies, customized footwear, and proactive foot care programs, are crucial for improving outcomes for diabetic patients. Ensuring access to such solutions will empower individuals to maintain their mobility, enhance their overall well-being, and improve their quality of life. Ultimately, this research aims to equip patients with the tools they need to manage their condition more effectively and prevent serious complications associated with DFUs.

9.3 Challenges and Future Scope

9.3.1 Enhancing Computational Models

In recent decades, significant advancements have been made in finite element modeling (FEM) of the diabetic foot, a crucial area of research given the high risk of complications associated with diabetes. However, despite these developments, there remains a substantial need for further refinement to achieve precise analyses and more reliable clinical outcomes. Specifically, there is an ongoing demand for innovative techniques that can create detailed three-dimensional (3D) foot models, which effectively capture the intricate anatomical structures, including muscles, tendons, ligaments, and soft tissues, that are vital to understanding the diabetic foot's mechanics. One promising approach to developing these comprehensive 3D models involves the combined use of computed tomography (CT) and magnetic resonance imaging (MRI). CT scans are particularly valuable for their ability to provide detailed images of bone structure, revealing the geometry and alignment of the skeletal components within the foot. However, one of the limitations of CT imaging lies in its reduced ability to accurately demonstrate the locations and orientations of soft-tissue structures, such as tendons and ligaments. This limitation arises from the way X-rays penetrate soft tissues, often leading to diminished resolution and clarity in images of these critical components. In contrast, MRI technology stands out in its capacity to provide superior detail regarding soft tissue and muscular anatomical features.

MRI scans can visualize the complex interplay of muscles, tendons, and ligaments with high contrast, allowing for a more comprehensive understanding of the foot's anatomy. While MRI is renowned for these advantages, its higher cost and relative availability compared to CT scans can limit its widespread use in certain clinical environments. By integrating imagery from both CT and MRI, researchers can develop enhanced 3D foot models that reflect a high level of biofidelity. These sophisticated models are not only beneficial for visualizing anatomical structures but also play a crucial role in predicting the mechanical behavior of the diabetic foot. Improved understanding of this biomechanical behavior can ultimately facilitate the creation of more effective, personalized treatment plans tailored to the specific needs of diabetic patients, thus promoting better clinical outcomes and reducing the risk of serious complications.

To ensure the reliability and accuracy of FE simulations, it is crucial to implement robust calibration and validation techniques tailored to the developed FE model. Calibration is a systematic process that involves validating experimental data against various material constitutive models. This is done to ascertain that the material constants selected during calibration yield a mechanical response in the FE model that closely resembles the behavior observed in experimental data. Specifically, when calibrating a full-scale FE foot model, it is imperative to adjust the parameters to fine-tune the model's response, ensuring that it accurately represents the biomechanics observed during gait movement analysis. A vital aspect of this calibration is conducting a mesh convergence study. This study verifies that the accuracy of the FE findings is maintained as the number of meshed elements increases. A well-conducted mesh convergence study ensures that the results are not influenced by the mesh quality, thereby enhancing the reliability of the simulation outcomes. Furthermore, an exhaustive evaluation of the interfacial characteristics among various components of the foot model is essential for establishing the upper and lower limits of output responses. These characteristics include the interactions between different tissues, specifically bone-bone, bone-muscle, muscle–tendon, and muscle-soft tissue interactions.

Given the challenges in obtaining experimental measurements of these interfacial properties across various regions of the foot, an advanced methodology must be employed for their estimation. One effective approach to investigate the effects of interfacial characteristics on the finite element analysis results is to perform foot model simulations under two different scenarios. In the first scenario, the interfacial properties can be assumed to be completely fixed, creating a baseline for comparison. In the second scenario, simulations can incorporate slip interfacial values, allowing for a more realistic representation of tissue interactions. By analyzing the outcomes from these two sets of simulations, researchers can identify the upper and lower limits of results and explore a range of outcomes that reflect more realistic interfacial characteristics. When simulating the effects of diabetic neuropathy on plantar pressures, it is crucial to utilize both kinematic and kinetic data derived from both healthy and diabetic neuropathic FE models. A comprehensive validation process must accompany these simulations, which includes a meticulous comparison between the experimental plantar pressures and those predicted by the FE models. This validation process is vital for identifying any discrepancies and addressing them to refine the models effectively. Discrepancies may arise, especially from patient-specific computational models that might produce pressures and strains that significantly deviate from the actual conditions. Such deviations can be attributed to variations in foot structure, loading patterns, the underlying diabetic condition, or the mode of ulceration. In such instances, conducting a detailed analysis to compare simulated results against real-world data is paramount. By integrating the simulated pressures into a broader analytical framework, our understanding of how diabetic neuropathy affects the foot can be significantly enhanced. This, in turn, opens up new avenues for improving treatment options and interventions for individuals affected by this condition. Therefore, systematically incorporating these techniques for calibrating, verifying, and validating the FE model not only enhances its reliability and accuracy but also enriches our comprehension of the foot's overall biomechanics during gait analysis.

The current methodology for developing computational foot models predominantly relies on utilizing CT and MRI data from specific individuals. While this approach provides valuable insights, it poses significant challenges when attempting to create a foot model that accurately represents a broader population. The limitations of the existing framework inhibit its applicability across diverse demographics, which is crucial for widespread use in fields such as orthopedics, prosthetics, and footwear design. To address this issue, future research should focus on creating a novel transformation technique aimed at efficiently modifying a reference foot model to align with individual foot geometries. This approach must take into account a variety of anthropometric factors, including but not limited to foot sizes and classifications such as normal arches versus flatfoot. By incorporating innovative transformation functions, such as scaling factors derived from experimental data and virtual motion capture markers placed strategically on the foot, this technique promises to adapt the reference model without losing the intricacies of individual variations. Implementing this transformation method could lead to considerable time savings compared to the traditional, labor-intensive process of reconstructing three-dimensional foot models directly from CT or MRI scans. Not only would this enhance efficiency in model generation, but it would also facilitate the creation of a more inclusive computational foot model that reflects the diversity found in the general population. Moreover, Fig. 9.1 illustrates the comprehensive stages involved in the development of computational foot models, highlighting their respective limitations and existing gaps in research. This visualization underscores the need for more research in this area. The work proposed is a pivotal step toward developing a robust and versatile computational foot model that can be utilized in various applications, including medical diagnostics, the design of prosthetic devices, and the advancement of ergonomic footwear, ultimately improving outcomes in health and comfort for individuals across different populations.

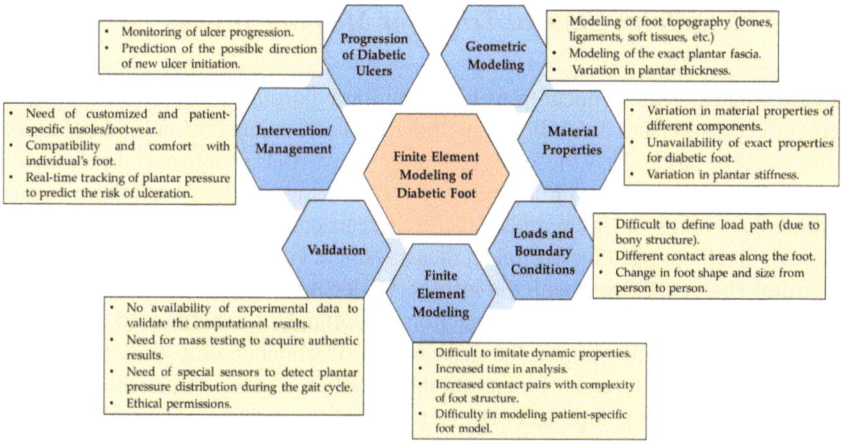

Fig. 9.1 FEM stages for diabetic foot modelling and their respective challenges. *Reproduced with permission from IOP Science* [3]

9.3.2 Integration of Smart Insoles with Mobile Health Platforms

The integration of smart pressure measurement insoles with mobile health applications stands to significantly transform patient care, particularly in the area of podiatric health, by enabling continuous and comprehensive monitoring of foot condition. These advanced insoles are equipped with sensors that precisely track pressure distribution in real time, delivering crucial insights into a patient's gait, weight-bearing patterns, and overall foot dynamics. This detailed data collection is invaluable for providing patients with timely and actionable feedback regarding their foot health. For individuals with diabetes or other conditions that impair circulation and sensory function, such insights can be especially life changing. By enabling early detection of abnormal pressure points or gait irregularities, these smart insoles can help prevent serious complications, such as foot ulcers or infections, which are common in at-risk populations. To facilitate widespread adoption and maximize the effectiveness of this technology, it is essential to create user-friendly mobile applications with intuitive interfaces. Such designs should prioritize ease of interaction, ensuring that patients can effortlessly access their data, receive alerts, and understand their health metrics without requiring extensive technical knowledge. This innovation represents a significant advancement in the management of diabetic foot health and leverages proactive health monitoring to not only enhance the effectiveness of smart insoles but also empower patients to take control of their well-being. By focusing on patient-centric design and real-time data utilization, we can usher in a new era of preventive care that significantly improves outcomes for individuals at risk of foot-related complications.

9.3.3 Long-Term Clinical Trials for Modular Insoles

Conducting extensive clinical trials is crucial for a thorough evaluation of the long-term effectiveness and durability of modular insoles designed for individuals at risk of foot ulcers, particularly those with diabetes. These trials should encompass a wide range of key outcomes, with a primary focus on assessing how well these insoles reduce plantar pressure, a significant factor that can lead to the occurrence or reoccurrence of ulcers. In addition to clinical measures, it is vital to gather patient feedback regarding their experience with the insoles. Understanding comfort levels of participants, ease of use, and overall satisfaction is essential, as adherence to using these insoles can significantly impact the success of the treatment protocol. Factors such as lifestyle compatibility, ease of integration into daily routines, and patient motivation play crucial roles in compliance. By systematically collecting comprehensive data over an extended period, researchers will be able to paint a clearer picture of both the advantages and potential limitations of these customized insoles [15]. This research will help identify which specific features are most beneficial for preventing diabetic foot ulceration and inform future design improvements to enhance patient outcomes. Ultimately, the insights gained from these trials can contribute to better clinical practices and improved quality of life for patients susceptible to foot complications.

References

1. Gupta S, Singh G, Chanda A (2021) Prediction of diabetic foot ulcer progression: a computational study. Biomed Phys Eng Express 7:065020
2. Gupta S et al (2023) Diabot: development of a diabetic foot pressure tracking device. J 6, 32–47
3. Singh G, Chanda A (2024) Finite element modeling of diabetic foot: a state-of-the-art review. Eng Res Express 6:012507
4. Owings TM et al (2009) Plantar pressures in diabetic patients with foot ulcers which have remained healed. Diabet Med 26:1141–1146
5. Fernando ME et al (2016) Plantar pressures are higher in cases with diabetic foot ulcers compared to controls despite a longer stance phase duration. BMC Endocr Disord 16:51
6. Singh G, Gupta S, Chanda A (2021) Biomechanical modelling of diabetic foot ulcers: A computational study. J Biomech 127:110699
7. Singh G, Chanda A (2022) Biomechanical modeling of progressive wound healing: A computational study. Biomed. Eng. Adv. 4:100055
8. Maghami E et al (2021) Fracture behavior of human cortical bone: Role of advanced glycation end-products and microstructural features. J Biomech 125:110600
9. Sáez P, Alastrué V, Peña E, Doblaré M, Martínez MA (2011) Anisotropic microsphere-based approach to damage in soft fibered tissue. Biomech Model Mechanobiol. 2011 115 11, 595–608
10. Bates JHT, Ma B (2013) A progressive rupture model of soft tissue stress relaxation. Ann Biomed Eng 416 41, 1129–1138
11. Li W (2016) Damage models for soft tissues: a survey. J Med Biol Eng. 363 36, 285–307
12. Bose D, Singh G, Gupta S, Chanda A (2024) Development of a novel customized insole for effective pressure offloading in diabetic patients. Prosthesis 6:341–356
13. Singh G, Bose D, Chanda A (2025) Development and testing of a novel diabetic orthosis for plantar pressure reduction. Facta Univ Ser Mech Eng. https://doi.org/10.22190/FUME240725044S

14. Chhikara K, Singh G, Gupta S, Chanda A (2022) Progress of additive manufacturing in fabrication of foot orthoses for diabetic patients: A review. Ann 3D Print Med 8, 100085
15. Gefen A, Megido-Ravid M, Azariah M, Itzchak Y, Arcan M (2001) Integration of plantar soft tissue stiffness measurements in routine MRI of the diabetic foot. Clin Biomech 16:921–925

MIX
Papier aus verantwortungsvollen Quellen
Paper from responsible sources
FSC® C105338

FSC
www.fsc.org

If you have any concerns about our products,
you can contact us on
ProductSafety@springernature.com

In case Publisher is established outside the EU,
the EU authorized representative is:
Springer Nature Customer Service Center GmbH
Europaplatz 3, 69115 Heidelberg, Germany

Printed by Libri Plureos GmbH
in Hamburg, Germany